Helping Schoolchildren with Chronic Health Conditions

The Guilford Practical Intervention in the Schools Series

Kenneth W. Merrell, Series Editor

Helping Students Overcome Depression and Anxiety: A Practical Guide
Kenneth W. Merrell

Emotional and Behavioral Problems of Young Children:
Effective Interventions in the Preschool and Kindergarten Years
Gretchen A. Gimpel and Melissa L. Holland

Conducting School-Based Functional Behavioral Assessments:
A Practitioner's Guide
T. Steuart Watson and Mark W. Steege

Executive Skills in Children and Adolescents: A Practical Guide
to Assessment and Intervention
Peg Dawson and Richard Guare

Responding to Problem Behavior in Schools:
The Behavior Education Program
Deanne A. Crone, Robert H. Horner, and Leanne S. Hawken

Resilient Classrooms: Creating Healthy Environments for Learning
Beth Doll, Steven Zucker, and Katherine Brehm

Helping Schoolchildren with Chronic Health Conditions:
A Practical Guide
Daniel L. Clay

Helping Schoolchildren
with Chronic Health Conditions

A Practical Guide

DANIEL L. CLAY

gp

THE GUILFORD PRESS
New York   London

© 2004 The Guilford Press
A Division of Guilford Publications, Inc.
72 Spring Street, New York, NY 10012
www.guilford.com

Printed in Canada

This book is printed on acid-free paper.

Last digit is print number: 9 8 7 6 5 4 3 2 1

Library of Congress Cataloging-in-Publication Data

Clay, Daniel, 1967–
    Helping schoolchildren with chronic health conditions: a practical guide / by Daniel L. Clay.
        p. cm.—(The Guilford practical intervention in the schools series)
Includes bibliographical references and index.
    ISBN 1-59385-043-3 (pbk.)
    1. School health services—United States—Handbooks, manuals, etc. 2. School children—Health and hygiene—United States—Handbooks, manuals, etc. 3. Chronically ill children—Medical care—United States—Handbooks, manuals, etc. I. Title. II. Series.
    LB3409.U5C53 2004
    371.71—dc22
                                                                                      2003027150

About the Author

Daniel L. Clay, PhD, is a licensed psychologist and Associate Professor of Counseling Psychology and Director of the Counseling Psychology Program at the University of Iowa. His research and clinical interests address children's health concerns, with a specific focus on children with chronic medical conditions and their families. Dr. Clay has authored numerous research articles in professional journals, book chapters, and books. He also has been recognized by the American Psychological Association for his excellence in research. Dr. Clay has extensive clinical experience working with children who have ill health or disability, and he is an advocate for such children and their families in medical and educational settings in several states.

Acknowledgments

I wish to acknowledge many people for their assistance in the completion of this book. Most importantly, I wish to thank Kenneth Merrell, editor of The Guilford Practical Intervention in the Schools Series, for his support and encouragement from the first ideas about this book to the final stages of manuscript completion. I also thank Chris Jennison of The Guilford Press for his patience and support during my work on the book. Several people made valuable contributions to the book through various activities. Dennis Harper was instrumental in the development of the ideas and structure of the book and contributed material for Chapter 2. Raelynn Maloney and Jami Gross were very helpful in the development of Chapters 6 and 7 and were consequently added as coauthors of those chapters for their contributions. I wish to also thank Julie Kettmann and Nicole Hochhausen for their assistance in developing materials for Chapter 2. Finally, I also greatly appreciate the assistance of Matt Raw, who demonstrated great patience with me during the numerous revisions of the book.

Contents

List of Tables, Figures, Worksheets, and Handouts

TABLES

FIGURES

WORKSHEETS

HANDOUTS

1

Introduction

WHY IS THIS BOOK IMPORTANT?

Due to advances in technology, more and more children who have significant health problems survive and participate in school. Likewise, changes in the health care environment have emphasized keeping children out of the hospital. As a result of these changes, an increasing number of the estimated 10–15% of children who will experience a chronic health problem are attending school on a regular basis. Although attending school is clearly beneficial for children with health problems, their presence in the schools has placed additional responsibilities on school personnel. In fact, federal legislation mandates schools' responsibility for addressing the needs of these children, when problems associated with the illness negatively affect the educational experience. School teachers, counselors, psychologists, administrators, and nurses are not only expected to work with children who have health problems, they are also responsible for providing an optimal educational environment for them. These responsibilities may include making curricular accommodations, monitoring health symptoms, collaborating with physicians and other health care providers, and supervising or even providing certain aspects of medical treatment while the children are in school. Not only are these expectations of school personnel demanding, little information is available to help them deal with the often complex and difficult issues that may arise. The purpose of this book is to help school personnel with these critical issues by providing practical strategies that are helpful in fulfilling school-based responsibilities to children with health problems and their families.

Over the last 10 years, I have noticed a shift in the responsibilities of pediatric psychologists as well. Responsibilities have increasingly shifted toward consulting with school personnel and families to help deal with all of the issues that arise within the school setting. Pediatric psychologists are increasingly working with parents to help their children to succeed in school. Likewise, they are working with school personnel to provide the specific information needed to create optimal learning environments using the limited resources afforded to school personnel. The following three examples of students with health concerns illustrate the difficult and complex issues that typically arise.

Example 1: Carol

Carol is an 8-year-old girl with insulin-dependent diabetes who is in the second grade. She requires daily insulin shots in school and occasional snacks when her blood sugar gets low. She has an individualized education plan (IEP) that outlines the responsibility of school personnel to help control and monitor her diabetes. Her control of the diabetes is often unpredictable, and she occasionally misses school during brief hospitalizations.

Questions/issues

1. How does Carol's diabetes affect her learning?
2. What do school personnel tell the other children when they ask why Carol gets a snack during class and they don't?
3. How do school personnel handle Carol's school absences?
4. What strategies can school personnel use to help Carol monitor her own blood sugar?
5. How can school personnel best communicate with Carol's parents and physician?

Example 2: Ryan

Ryan is a 14-year-old boy with a long history of severe asthma. He is small for his age and socially delayed due to his extended absences from school. He carries an inhaler to control his asthma attacks. Ryan is often required to sit out during physical education class and other activities that may expose him to dust or chemicals (e.g., field trips and science lab). He is the last to be selected for class activities, and other children often tease him. His teacher's concerns are many:

Questions/issues

1. What should school personnel do if Ryan has an asthma attack?
2. What do school personnel do when other children pick on Ryan or he is chosen last for a team?
3. How should school personnel handle his absence from a valuable class experience?
4. Who monitors his medications? What are their effects on his behavior and learning?
5. How can school personnel help Ryan to fit in better socially?
6. Is there anything that school personnel can do to help prevent his asthma attacks?
7. Who should school personnel talk to if his asthma seems to be getting worse?

Example 3: Elisa

Elisa is a 12-year-old girl who has been receiving treatment for cancer. She has been absent from school for nearly 2 months and has recently been attending school for half-days. She is often sleepy, whiny, and fatigued in school, and she cries often, asking to go home. Her parents are firm in their decision to keep her in school for the half-days. Elisa's parents are also keeping private the information regarding their daughter's course of treatment and prognosis. Her teacher has the following concerns:

Questions/issues

1. How much emphasis should school personnel place on Elisa's completion of her assignments?
2. What do school personnel tell other children when they ask if Elisa is going to die?
3. What can school personnel do when she cries and whines about her pain?
4. How do school personnel handle her parents, who seem to have unreasonable expectations?
5. What activities should school personnel insist Elisa participate in?
6. How can school personnel help her talk to the other children about her condition?

BRIEF OVERVIEW OF BOOK CONTENT

With this overview of the issues addressed in this book, let's turn briefly to a discussion of health and illness concepts as they relate to the educational system. Although prevention of sickness or illness is obviously important, and I recognize the importance of health promotion and prevention programs in the school environment, I focus on the remedial aspects of illness that include recovery from acute illness or injury as well as the long-term implications of living with chronic medical or health conditions. By this I mean conditions that require some form of periodic or ongoing medical treatment, which may have an immediate and/or enduring impact on a child and his or her family within the educational context. Such illnesses include diabetes, cancer, seizure disorders, pain (stomach, headache, joints, etc.), asthma, juvenile arthritis, blood disorders (e.g., hemophilia), and tic disorders.

There are many other medical disorders that are beyond the scope of this book. However, many of the same issues discussed in this book also apply to these illnesses or conditions. For example, school support personnel are faced with many of the same issues when children have conditions such as cerebral palsy or brain injury. Likewise, many of the strategies and issues included in this book apply when working with children who have depression, anxiety, or attention-deficit/hyperactivity disorder. These conditions are addressed more directly in other books in The Guilford Practical Intervention in the Schools series.

In addition to focusing on the specific issues and problems that arise from medical illnesses, I also discuss strategies that promote overall health and wellness within the school environment. Children obviously must have adequate nutrition, exercise, and social stimulation within the school setting to provide an optimal environment for their learning and social development. Although I focus on detailed and specific strategies, it is important to keep in mind that my broad goals include helping school personnel provide optimal learning environments and maximize student participation in learning. To that end, I address medical, social, educational, and developmental issues that interact to influence the school environment for children with health concerns. For example, I suggest practical strategies on how to manage teasing that may occur to ensure that children feel safe and valued. Although feeling safe and valued may not, at first glance, seem to be related to health issues, it is important to address such issues to ensure that personnel are optimally prepared to handle all issues that may arise for these children.

PURPOSE OF THIS BOOK

This book is designed to be a resource guide for school personnel, including administrators, counselors, teachers, school psychologists, and social workers, for children and their parents, and for health care professionals. The material in this book is based on scientific research and many years of experience working with children who have health problems. However, I have avoided the use of jargon and technical language that often prevents the application of scientific research and experience to school-based interventions. Information covered includes the common issues associated with specific health conditions, practical information to assess children's needs, specific strategies for dealing with associated issues, specific interventions, and tips for minimizing the negative impact of the health condition on children's ability to attend and benefit from school. The overall emphasis is on providing practical strategies for coping with health concerns and issues in the classroom and school environment.

FORMAT OF THIS BOOK

The format of this book lends itself well to use as a resource manual. Lists of specific strategies, tables of checklists, handouts, and assessment instruments are available for photocopying and use with individual cases. Issues and specific health conditions are cross-referenced for easy use. For example, if you have a student with cancer who is being teased by other children, you can look at Chapter 2 to learn about the issues associated with cancer, and/or Chapter 5 to see how to deal with teasing and exclusion by other children. Likewise, Chapter 5 can be checked to see if, when, and how to tell other children about the cancer, as well as specific strategies for how to approach the sensitive discussion (e.g., should the child with cancer be present during the discussion?). Since schools have a legal responsibility to provide appropriate services, Chapter 3 examines the legal history and Chapter 4 covers the development of educational plans to address the individual educational needs of these children, as dictated by law. The last chapter integrates and applies the important issues discussed in earlier chapters and provides an example of the application of the strategies to a specific case.

Main Objectives of This Book

This book is designed to help you:

1. Understand common childhood health problems
2. Understand how health problems impact the child in the school environment
3. Utilize methods and strategies for assessing the impact of health problems in the school environment
4. Facilitate collaboration among health care professionals, families, and educators
5. Learn strategies for assisting and intervening with children who have health problems
6. Develop individualized education plans (IEPs) and 504 plans to address the individual needs of children with chronic illness

CONCLUDING COMMENTS

In the last several decades substantial progress has been made in treating medical illnesses in children. Consequently, the numbers of children surviving with a chronic medical problem have risen sharply, and these children are now attending school. These trends, combined with legislation mandating schools to address the multiple needs of children with chronic illness, have left educators with huge responsibilities and, oftentimes, inadequate resources to handle those responsibilities. Chronic illnesses frequently impact the children's ability to attend and benefit from traditional education. Yet information specifically designed to help educators deal with such issues is severely lacking. This book attempts to address this need by providing practical information that can be readily applied to individual cases. Several reproducible worksheets and handouts at the end of Chapters 4–7 are designed to provide easy reference materials. I also demonstrate concepts through the use of case examples.

2

Overview of Common Health Conditions

CHAPTER OBJECTIVES

The number of health conditions affecting children in the school environment is in the hundreds. Reviewing all of these illnesses here would be impossible and impractical. Consequently, I have reviewed the high-frequency medical disorders and health problems that you are most likely to encounter as well as health conditions that have lower incidence but which may still have a significant influence within the school environment. I have chosen to exclude developmental disorders, disabling conditions such as cerebral palsy and spina bifida, as well as other genetic conditions such as Down syndrome (although many of the issues discussed in this book may be helpful with these conditions).

I briefly summarize each condition or illness, its important characteristics, and the medical treatment issues. This overview is intended to provide the baseline knowledge that is necessary to best serve these children in the school environment. I then discuss in more detail the potential impact the given condition may have on the school environment, including attendance, participation in activities, necessary treatments, and effects on learning. The main characteristics, impact on education, and additional Web-based resources for each illness are listed in a table. To summarize these objectives:

- To identify and summarize characteristics of high-incidence and low-incidence chronic medical conditions
- To discuss the potential impact of these illnesses on school attendance and performance
- To identify additional Web-based resources for further information on each illness

HIGH-INCIDENCE CONDITIONS

Diabetes

Diabetes mellitus is a disorder of carbohydrate metabolism involving the imbalance of supply and demand for insulin in the body. This condition can affect all parts of the body. The cause is currently unknown, but there is a tendency for it to occur in families. Diabetes can also occur as a result of other conditions and infections. The condition that affects young children, juvenile-onset, type I—also called insulin-dependent diabetes mellitus, or IDMM— occurs in about 15–20 children out of 100,000 under the age of 20 (Daneman & Frank, 1996). Type I diabetes requires insulin injections or shots and can be difficult to control. Type II diabetes in children and adolescents is usually associated with obesity and can be treated with pills and diet. Currently there is no cure for diabetes mellitus. Rather, treatment is directed toward controlling the levels of blood sugar (glucose) in the blood and preventing long-term complications (e.g., skin lesions, nerve damage, kidney problems, visual problems). The treatment issues are not simple, especially for active and growing children; compliance with blood checking, medication, diet, and exercise is a challenging task and must be done in a coordinated fashion. Treatment or management consists of (1) monitoring blood sugar using a glucometer (an automated finger-sticking device for measuring glucose levels in the blood), (2) adjusting insulin amounts, (3) administering or overseeing insulin shots, watching daily diet, and monitoring the amount of overall daily exercise. The salient goal is to avoid hypoglycemia: too much insulin in the blood for the amount of sugar. Hypoglycemia or insulin shock may make individuals feel weak, nervous, sweaty, and produce mood changes. In contrast, *diabetic coma* occurs when there is too much sugar in the blood; initially, individuals may appear confused, drowsy, and rather sleepy. These changes in behavior or mood are important when monitoring diabetes in children and youth. The family, physician, and school nurse are excellent resources for information in this area and should be consulted regarding individual issues and health care for each student. Treatment for type I and II diabetes has different demands. Some children need to monitor their blood sugar and administer shots at school, and the school nurse is the logical assistant, if available. A private setting for the student is helpful, along with a storage location for medications. The student with type II, which is usually associated with obesity, needs special support regarding weight management and self-esteem issues.

Diabetes mellitus is a "hidden disability" whose symptoms are not always present or visible. Attitudes of the family, peers, and the child with diabetes are often the key factors in successfully coping with its ongoing management. In many instances the school program will provide an individualized health plan (IHP) for the student, in cooperation with the local doctor, the family, and school personnel. This plan needs to (1) manage the schedule of snacks, activities, and eating on field trips; (2) deal with potential blood sugar fluctuations (e.g., maintain a supply of glucose tablets, juice, raisins, and crackers) and establish prearranged communication with the teacher regarding the child's needs; (3) accommodate requests for more water, trips to the bathroom, etc.; (4) address lunchroom eating issues; (5) address special circumstances, such as classroom parties with their typically sugar-laden foods; and (6) provide a list of medical and family phone numbers for special needs or emergencies.

TABLE 2.1. Major Characteristics, Educational Concerns and Complications, and Additional Resources for Students with Diabetes

Major characteristics	Educational concerns and complications	Additional resources

• Hypoglycemia, or insulin shock
  • Weak
  • Nervous
  • Sweaty
  • Mood changes
• Hyperglycemia, or to much sugar in the blood
  • Confused
  • Drowsy
  • Sleepy
  • Thirsty
  • Frequent urination
	• Observe changes in mood or behavior.
	• Hyperglycemia can lead to diabetic coma, which can be life threatening.
	• Hypoglycemia can lead to passing out.
	• Some children need to monitor blood sugar levels and receive insulin shots.
	• Manage the schedule of lunch, snacks, and activities.
	• Deal with low blood sugar (e.g., maintains a supply of glucose tablets, juice, raisins, and crackers).
	• Accommodate students' requests for more water or more trips to the bathroom; may signal hyperglycemia.
	• May need special foods for lunch room and classroom parties.
		• American Diabetes Association: *http://www.diabetes.org*
		• Lifeclinic: *http://www.lifeclinic.com/focus/diabetes/childrenteen_main.asp*
		• Children with Diabetes: *http://www.childrenwithdiabetes.com/d_0q_200.htm*
		• Diabetes Living: *http://www.diabetesliving.com/kids/kds_schl.htm*

Diabetes mellitus can have an impact on learning activities and social interactions. Direct effects on learning can be related to mood and attentional issues associated with blood sugar and insulin variations. However, these possible reasons should be carefully considered along with the other more common situational reasons for such variations in all children and youth. We want to avoid becoming overly vigilant and overinterpreting every slight slump or mistake. When in doubt, ask the child and check with the parent and the doctor. Indirect effects of diabetes include difficult social and interpersonal factors: Children, especially adolescents, often feel too different from many of their peers and may react with noncompliance over health management issues. Occasionally, some counseling may be needed. Future concerns about long-term implications often surface during adolescence, and there is a need for open and honest communication of information, usually provided by other local health professionals or the family. Table 2.1 summarizes the main characteristics, impact on education, and additional resources for dealing with students with diabetes in the classroom.

Asthma

Asthma is the most common of chronic childhood illnesses, affecting nearly 5 million children under the age of 18 in the United States. Asthma is a respiratory condition characterized by difficulty breathing, wheezing and coughing, shortness of breath, chest tightness, and fatigue. In general, asthma is more common in boys, African Americans, and people living in poverty. Environmental substances such as dust, pollens, smoke, dander from pets, molds, and any other airborne substances that can be breathed into the lungs can trigger asthma attacks. The condition is often sporadic and variable in intensity. Treatment for asthma varies depending on severity and can include both preventive measures, such as minimizing exposure to triggers, and medical measures, such as medication. Treatments can range from self-administered inhalers to the regular use of nebulizer treatments (a machine that turns medication into vapor to be inhaled) to hospitalization. Most children with asthma require some form of treatment during school hours. Most likely, children need to carry an inhaler to self-administer medications when they feel the first signs of an impending asthma attack. Although the long-term prognosis for asthma is good in most cases, asthma attacks can be fatal. Consequently, it is very important for such instances to be treated as medical emergencies.

Asthma may have a negative impact on the school environment in a number of ways. Although there are no documented cognitive deficits or learning disabilities associated with asthma, side effects of some medications may cause impairment in memory and attention, hyperactivity, anxiety and depression, and drowsiness. Children with asthma may have higher rates of absenteeism, which is likely to have an adverse impact on their school achievement and social development. Furthermore, limiting a child's activities with classmates (e.g., physical education, science experiments) can have negative social implications, especially if he or she feels ashamed of, embarrassed by, or angry about being excluded. Children with asthma usually need continual monitoring and access to treatment within the school environment, making it necessary for teachers, administrators, and school nurses to be educated about asthma and to remain involved with the child. Older school buildings, with their high levels of dust and mold, are often problematic for children with asthma and may contribute to their health problems. Table 2.2 summarizes the main characteristics, impact on education, and additional resources for dealing with students with asthma in the classroom.

TABLE 2.2. Major Characteristics, Educational Concerns and Complications, and Additional Resources for Students with Asthma

Major characteristics	Educational concerns and complications	Additional resources
• Wheezing • Coughing • Fatigue • Chest tightness • Can be triggered by dusty environmental conditions (e.g., mold, dust, chemicals). • Medication needed.	• Medications may cause irritability and cognitive difficulties. • Continual monitoring required. • Children may need to take frequent trips to nurses office or store inhalers in the classroom. • Attacks can be life threatening.	• American Academy of Allergy Asthma and Immunology: *www.aaaai.org* • SafeChild.net: *http://www.safechild.net/for_professionals/asthma.html* • Calgary Allergy Network: *http://www.calgaryallergy.ca/Articles/teacherast.html* • Sniffles & Sneezes: *http://www.allergyasthma.com/archives/asthma04.html*

Juvenile Rheumatoid Arthritis

Juvenile rheumatoid arthritis (JRA) is a chronic illness characterized by inflammation of the joints. Arthritis is typically seen as a disease that affects the aging population and may come as a surprise to people unaware that children can also have the disease. JRA is estimated to affect nearly 200,000 children in the United States under the age of 18. The disease is two to three times more likely to occur in girls than boys and appears to be unrelated to ethnic or socioeconomic groups. The onset of this type of arthritis can occur as early as infancy, with most cases diagnosed between the ages of 1 and 4 or between the ages of 8 and 12 (Cassidy & Petty, 1995). There are three subtypes of JRA: pauciarticular, polyarticular, and systemic. The details of the differences between the subtypes are not relevant for our purposes; in general, the three types range in severity from least severe (pauciarticular) to most severe (systemic). Symptoms include stiff, swollen, and painful joints, limited in range of movement, as well as fever and rash. Other health problems associated with JRA include enlarged lymph nodes, impairment of vision, and inflammation of the sac around the heart (which can be life threatening). JRA is often unpredictable; it can go into remission, never to return, recur or flare in severity without known cause, or simply continue to cause chronic pain and disability indefinitely. Although disfigurement can occur, most children do not experience permanent joint damage. However, about 10% of children with JRA enter adulthood with significant limits on functional capacity, and 15–30% of children with the pauciarticular subtype and eye involvement experience blindness (Cassidy & Petty, 1995). Treatment for JRA includes limiting activities, engaging in specialized exercises, and taking medications. Most treatments are carried out at home or school, although hospitalization may be needed in cases of severe disease activity, when intravenous medications are necessary. Typically, steroids, nonsteroidal anti-inflammatory drugs, or high doses of aspirin are used for pain relief and to reduce swelling.

JRA can have a significant impact on the child in the educational environment, especially during episodes of severe disease activity. The most frequent limitations involve activities that require bodily movement, such as writing, participating in physical education, getting from class to class in a limited time period, and sitting in the same position (i.e., at a desk) for an extended period of time. Involvement of the joints in the hands may also influence such self-care activities as eating and dressing, although this is less frequent than limitations in gross motor activities such as running and walking. It may be necessary to allow a child with JRA to stretch and exercise when needed during the school day, although contact sports and vigorous activities (such as running and jumping) are often limited. Likewise, a child with JRA may need more time to get from one location to another, particularly if it is necessary to climb stairs. There are no cognitive or learning disabilities associated with JRA, although some medication side effects may become problematic. Limited vision will be a significant factor for children with the pauciarticular subtype who also have eye involvement. These children may also experience excessive absences from school, the number, timing, and length of which are often unpredictable, given the unpredictability of the illness. In nearly all cases, children with active JRA need special accommodations within the school environment. Table 2.3 summarizes the main character-

TABLE 2.3. Major Characteristics, Educational Concerns and Complications, and Additional Resources for Students with Juvenile Rheumatoid Arthritis

Major characteristics	Educational concerns and complications	Additional resources
• Inflammation of the joints • Pain and stiffness • Limited range of movement • Unpredictable disease course; periods of inflammation and pain can have fast onset. • Impaired vision for some.	• Limits on some activities, such as writing, running, and maintaining the same position for extended periods of time. • When student is not experiencing inflammation, he or she can be encouraged to be active, but should refrain from high levels of physical activity to protect joints. • Excessive school absences are common. • Late arrival at school common; extreme stiffness, inflammation, and pain experienced in the morning. • Arrange seating so that student can stand and do stretching exercises inconspicuously throughout the day. • Allow extra time going from one place to another. • Due to pain and stiffness in hand joints, extra time may be needed for written tests; allow for oral exams. • May need to accommodate or assist student with joint supports, removable splints, or serial casts. • Student may experience anger and depression about the restrictions imposed by the disease. • Common side effect of anti-inflammatory drugs is nausea or need to eat frequently.	• Arthritis Foundation: *http://www.arthritis.org/resources/school_success.asp* • National Institute for Arthritis and Musculoskeletal and Skin Diseases: *http://www.niams.nih.gov/hi/topics/juvenile_arthritis/juvarthr.htm* • Arthritis Foundation: *http://www.arthritis.org/resources/classroom.asp*

istics, impact on education, and additional resources for dealing with students with JRA in the classroom.

Cancer

Cancer in children and adolescents most commonly manifests as one of the leukemias (blood cancer), lymphomas (cancer of the lymph system), or brain tumors. Cancer is generally understood to be an unchecked change in cell growth in various parts of the body, which often spreads (metastasizes) to other parts of the body. The cancer cells are often in competition with the body's normal cells for food and nutrients. Causes are related to toxic chemicals, tobacco use, some viruses, chronic irritations to the body, excessive sun, and hereditary predispositions. The good news is that childhood blood cancers, lymphomas, and brain tumors are all being treated with increasing success. Treatments are multimodal, often including chemotherapy, radiation (X rays), immunosuppressants, surgery, and bone marrow replacements. Goals include cure, life extension, prevention of the spread of cancer, and easing the pain and suffering.

Early diagnosis is often difficult because many cancer symptoms mimic those of other illnesses. If cancer is suspected, many pediatricians refer the young person to a medical center, which has teams of cancer specialists to confirm (or deny) the diagnosis and design a specific treatment plan, when needed. If the family lives some distance from the center, the local doctor often administers medicines and participates in the patient's care as well. Periodically the young person returns to the cancer center for reevaluation. Initial treatment may be intense, becoming more moderate if the young person responds adequately. It may be necessary to continue some form of treatment for several years. *Remission* and *relapse* (recurrence) are the terms used to describe the two main phases of the disease. A child is in remission when no evidence of cancer is detectable. Relapse refers to the return of the disease after improvement or a period of remission. If a complete remission continues for a number of years, the child's doctor may begin to think of the young person as "cured."

It is important to understand that the disease and the treatment can both produce physical changes in children, such as nausea, vomiting, and fatigue, which decrease energy levels and the ability to participate in a variety of school activities. Other possible changes, which are usually temporary, include weight gain or loss, mood swings, facial fullness and puffiness, problems with coordination, difficulty with fine and gross motor control, body marks resembling tattoos (indicating the sites of radiation therapy) and muscle weakness. Children with solid tumors may undergo surgical changes, such as amputations or scars. Hair loss is very common in many children undergoing chemotherapy, and perhaps to most of them, this is the more disturbing part of their treatment. The hair may fall out suddenly or over a period of weeks or months. It may grow back while the child is still receiving treatment but usually does not return to normal until after the chemotherapy has been completed. The young person might wear a wig, a hat, or a scarf to cover the hair loss. Any of these physical changes can result in teasing and, in some cases, rejection by peers, creating a reluctance to resume friendships, not to mention returning to school.

Young people with cancer can clearly benefit from attending school throughout their illness. However, doing so remains a challenge for them, the teacher, and their peers as well. Generally they feel better when they are productive in their role as learner and student for all the obvious reasons of participating in, and maintaining, normal routines. Frequent absences for medical reasons, occasional overprotection and/or overindulgence by parents may be a problem. Limitations on physical activity and social isolation tend to be common obstacles to regular school attendance by these children.

No matter how prepared we are, having a student with cancer in the classroom can be emotionally demanding and time consuming. There may be times when we feel somewhat overwhelmed by the situation. At these times it may be helpful to know that health profes-

TABLE 2.4. Major Characteristics, Educational Concerns and Complications, and Additional Resources for Students with Cancer

Major characteristics	Educational concerns and complications	Additional resources
• Disease and treatment cause nausea and vomiting • Fatigue • Mood swings • Difficulty with motor control • Muscle weakness due to treatment • Significant changes in appearance during treatment including temporary weight gain or loss, facial swelling, hair loss	• Anxiety • Emotional difficulties leading to behavior problems • Peer relationship difficulties resulting from social isolation, feared and rejected by peers • Teacher needs to educate peers about the child's situation so that they can be accepting and supportive. • Frustration related to school difficulties • Fatigue leading to decrease in energy levels to participate in activities • Excessive or extended absences • Assisting child in keeping up with schoolwork during hospital stays if possible • Teachers need a reintegration plan to help child best adjust when returns from extended hospital stay.	• American Cancer Society: *http://www.cancer.org/eprise/main/docroot/CRI/CRI_2x?sitearea=LRN&dt=7* • National Children's Cancer Society: • *http://www.children-cancer.com/links/index.html* • Band-Aides and Blackboards: *http://www.faculty.fairfield.edu/fleitas/healthed.html* • Candlelighter's Childhood Cancer Foundation: • *http://www.candlelighters.org/*

sionals who work with young people who have cancer are also subject to the same emotions and feel the same kinds of need for outside support.

In planning for the student's return to the classroom, some preliminary information is often very helpful. Contacting the parents to obtain the following information can be helpful:

- Specific type of cancer and how it is being treated.
- Potential side effects of treatment and effects on a child's behavior.
- Approximate time of upcoming treatments and procedures that will interfere with school attendance.
- Limitations, if any, on the student's activities.
- What the student knows about the illness.
- For younger students, what the family would like the classroom and school staff members to know.
- For adolescents, whether the student wishes to talk directly with the teachers about any of the above issues.

Despite improvement in survival rates, cancer in some children cannot be controlled and is ultimately fatal. Managing this discussion in a classroom can be a major challenge for teachers and children alike. When a student dies, classmates may express their grief in a variety of ways. Some are open about their feelings, whereas others may appear indifferent or very quiet. Such responses are normal variations of grief reactions. Feelings of loss should be acknowledged, and discussions should be open if the teacher is prepared to deal with these issues. It may be also useful to consult other school personnel, health personnel, or the school psychologist to assist in these discussions. Table 2.4 summarizes the main characteristics, impact on education, and additional resources for dealing with students with cancer in the classroom.

LOW-INCIDENCE CONDITIONS

Cystic Fibrosis

According to the Cystic Fibrosis Foundation, cystic fibrosis (CF) is a genetic condition found in an estimated 1 in 3,000 live births and is the most common lethal genetic disease in the U.S. white population. The illness is much less prevalent in Asian American and African American populations. Although CF is often a terminal disease, recent advances in treatment have extended the life expectancy to early adulthood. Although the disease is systemic, most symptoms observed by school personnel involve respiratory functioning. Respiratory symptoms of CF include wheezing, chronic and/or severe coughing with excessive secretions, and labored breathing. Other symptoms include retarded growth, fatigue, chronic diarrhea, delayed physical development, abdominal bloating, poor digestion and absorption of nutrition, and salty-tasting skin. Treatment for CF is highly specialized, intensive, and critical to prolonging the life of the child and providing the best quality of life possible. Treatments include (1) manual percussion of the chest cavity to encourage expulsion of excessive sticky secretions from lungs, (2) medications (oral and inhaled), and (3) special diets.

Because of the severity of CF and its progressive nature, children require extensive accommodations within the school environment. Extended and frequent absences may result from the health problems. Children with CF may be allowed to engage in only limited physical activities. Likewise, social isolation may occur as a result of absences due to the need for medical treatments, and peer rejection may surface because the child is seen as "different." Because CF may be fatal, children may experience high levels of anxiety around their possibly impending death. Any failure to meet peer accomplishments (academic or social) also produces anxiety and alienation. Although research on whether CF causes cognitive deficits has reported mixed findings, it is likely that the medications needed to treat this disease may affect cognitive capacity. It is essential for the child with CF to have an IEP. Teachers and other school personnel need to be aware of the educational and medical needs of the child. Academic progress will need to be monitored, and accommodations for extended absences may be necessary. The IEP should clarify responsibilities for any medical procedures that are necessary during the school day (see Chapter 4). As is usually the case with chronic illness in children, school personnel should maintain frequent and open communication with both the child's doctor and parent(s). Table 2.5

TABLE 2.5. Major Characteristics, Educational Concerns and Complications, and Additional Resources for Students with Cystic Fibrosis

Major characteristics	Educational concerns and complications	Additional resources

• Respiratory symptoms
  • Wheezing
  • Chronic and/or severe coughing
  • Excessive secretions
  • Labored breathing
• Other symptoms
  • Retarded growth
  • Fatigue
  • Chronic diarrhea
  • Delayed physical development
  • Abdominal bloating
  • Poor digestion and absorption of nutrition
  • Salty-tasting skin
	• Extended and frequent absences
	• Limited physical activities
	• Social isolation
	• Children may experience high anxiety and fear.
	• Children will require an IEP.
	• Some medical procedures may be necessary during school.
		• Canadian Cystic Fibrosis Foundation: *http:// www.cysticfibrosis.ca/pdf/ Teachers_Guide.pdf*
		• Cystic Fibrosis Foundation: *http://www.cff.org/living_with_ cf/teachers_guide.cfm*
		• Cystic Fibrosis Foundation: *http://www.cysticfibrosiswa.org/ schoolncf.html*

summarizes the main characteristics, impact on education, and additional resources for dealing with students with cystic fibrosis in the classroom.

Epilepsy/Seizures

Epilepsy is a physical condition caused by sudden and brief changes in brain-wave activity. When the cells of the brain are not working properly, a person's awareness, movements, and actions may be altered. These physical changes are called seizures, and epilepsy is sometimes called a seizure disorder. *Seizure* is a general term that is used to refer to temporary brain anomalies and altered awareness. Sometimes babies who have high fevers get seizures but do not have epilepsy, for example. Epilepsy affects people of all ages and races. About 40,000 cases a year are reported to begin in childhood, and about 1% of the total population now has epilepsy. In the majority of cases, no exact cause can be identified, but a variety of conditions has been linked to epilepsy onset: brain injuries, brain strokes, tumors in the brain, genetic conditions, lead poisoning, problems in the way the brain develops prenatally, certain illnesses such as brain infections or even severe cases of common diseases such as measles. In some ways, the incidence of epilepsy can be reduced by preventing seizure-producing illnesses such as head injuries. Epilepsy is not a contagious disease but it is an inherited condition, to some extent—most of the time, however, there is no family history of the condition at all.

There are different kinds of seizures. Generalized chronic seizures, also called grand mal seizures or convulsions, involve the whole brain. Sometimes the person falls to the ground, unconscious. The body stiffens and displays jerking movements. Breathing may get very slow and may even stop for a few minutes, causing the skin to turn somewhat blue. Sometimes bladder or bowel control is also lost during these seizures. When the person awakens, he or she may feel confused and sleepy. Only a very short period of recovery (5–10 minutes) is needed for some people, and most people go back to their normal activities after a half hour or so. If the seizure is somewhat prolonged, medical attention will be needed. In contrast, petit mal seizures look like daydreaming or blank spells. These are sometimes difficult to notice in children, but they do occur and can be problematical. A child having this kind of seizure is unaware of people and things around him or her for only a few seconds. These little seizures can happen so quickly that the child, and sometimes other people, may not even notice them. Sometimes they appear as blinking or chewing movements, turning of the head, or moving of the arms.

An aura is the experience of certain sensations just prior to a seizure (actually, the aura is the beginning of the seizure). People sometimes report feeling scared or sick to their stomach or having an odd smell or funny taste in their mouth. Most seizures do not seem to have any lasting effects. Many people with epilepsy have had dozens of seizures in their lives without any noticeable changes in their intelligence or their alertness. A seizure is very rarely a cause of death by itself, but there is danger involved, depending upon what the person is doing when the seizure strikes: riding a bike, swimming, or any activity where falling poses a danger. Death from seizures usually occurs only following a series of nonstop seizures that last for hours and hours and are not treated in a hospital.

It is important to remember that a person who is having a seizure cannot control his or her actions and is therefore not capable of carrying out a planned attack on someone or hurting anybody. Most people who have seizures are more likely to hurt themselves than anybody else.

Neurologists sometimes play very important roles in helping others treat seizures in children. To identify the presence of a seizure disorder, doctors use a very careful medical history obtained from parents and a brain test called an EEG (electroencephalogram). An electroencephalograph machine records brain waves and reveals how the brain is functioning. Sometimes special pictures of the brain—X rays, a CT (computerized tomography) scan, or an MRI (magnetic resonance imaging)—are taken to see if there are any other growth or other problems present. Seizures and epilepsy are treated with drugs, surgery, and sometimes a special diet. Drug therapy is the most common and successful form of treatment.

It is also important to remember that seizures or epilepsy is not the same as mental illness. Sometimes children who have epilepsy or seizures experience different kinds of emotions or feelings (e.g., anxiety, emotional arousal, or tingly sensations), some perhaps caused by a brief seizure in the part of the brain that controls emotions generally. It is best to report these kinds of emotional changes to the child's parents, and they can tell the doctor. Some people who have seizures may have some difficulty remembering things that happened recently, or remembering a sequence of actions or events. This difficulty might be due to the condition of seizures, the medicine, or other brain activity that co-occurs with the seizures. It is important to consider the possibility that some children with seizures may have some memory difficulties. A discussion of these issues with the parents and then a decision regarding the advisability of further evaluation by the school psychologist may help sort out some of these questions.

TABLE 2.6. Major Characteristics, Educational Concerns and Complications, and Additional Resources for Students with Epilepsy/Seizures

Major characteristics	Educational concerns and complications	Additional resources

• Chronic seizures
  • Also called *grand mal* seizures or *convulsions*.
  • Person may fall to ground and become unconscious.
  • Body stiffens.
  • Movements jerky.
  • Breathing slows and may stop, causing skin to turn somewhat blue.
  • Loss of bladder or bowel control may occur.
• Absence seizures
  • Also called *petit mal* seizures.
  • Look like daydreaming or blank spells.
  • May appear as blinking or chewing movements, turning of the head, or moving of the arms.
  • Aura (occasional feeling presaging a seizure)
  • Feeling scared or sick to their stomach.
  • Having an odd smell or funny taste in the mouth.
	• If seizures are prolonged, medical attention may be needed.
	• Most children can return to regular activities after a brief rest period.
	• Children may have memory difficulties.
	• Carefully review with parents and the child how they prefer the seizures to be addressed with other students.
		• Epilepsy Association Australia: *http://www.epilepsy.com.au/ epilepsy/epilepsyadult.nsf/ Content/Teachers*
		• Northeast Rehabilitation Health Network: *http:// www.northeastrehab.com/ Articles/seizurefaq.htm*
		• Alaska Rehabilitation Specialists: *http:// www.alaska.net/~drussell/ars/ e_teach1.html*

Children who have seizures in the classroom present a complicated challenge for their teachers, not only in regard to their management and assistance but as well from the numerous questions raised by their classmates. It is very important to obtain current and accurate information from the children's parents and the local doctor and to review it with a school health professional. Discussion of these issues in class is an especially sensitive concern and needs to be carefully reviewed with the child's parents and as well the child, as he or she becomes older. Many challenging attitudes still surround seizures and epilepsy, and the child's own self-esteem and attitudes are often affected as much (or more) by these factors as they are by the condition itself. Table 2.6 summarizes the main characteristics, impact on education, and additional resources for dealing with students who have epilepsy or other seizure disorders.

Stress-Related Conditions (Headache, Stomach Pain)

Stress is a feeling of discomfort that is experienced somewhat differently from one individual to another, whether children or adults. Additionally, constitutional factors, including gender and temperament, often play a significant role in how stress is perceived and handled. Children in school experience a variety of stresses that can be related to general school performance, poor grades, tests, scheduling changes, and so on. Home events can also affect children's performance in school. Stress is cumulative and progressive, and improved resources and coping skills are often necessary to reduce its effects. The important point is not to try to eliminate stress (an impossible task) but to look for ways to manage it and to be aware of the signs and symptoms of stress in children.

Symptoms of stress in preschool and young children may be difficult to distinguish from symptoms of minor illness. We need to be alert for signs of irritability, clinginess, nervousness, inattention, fearfulness, difficulties adapting to change in routine, and use of key words such as "sad" or "afraid." As children get older, their responses to stress may include more mood changes, isolation from peers, attention-seeking behaviors, school refusal, or changes in the quality of their schoolwork, and physical complaints such as headache, stomachache, or general body aches. Stress is often a frequent contributor to short tempers on the playground, fights in the lunchroom, or avoidance of classroom activities or school, in general.

Children who have experienced sudden or intense levels of stress may develop posttraumatic stress disorder (PTSD). In these cases the stress is often related to a specific event and appears to result in high levels of nervousness and general anxiety. Children who display high levels of nervousness, seemingly "out of the blue," probably should be referred to the counselor or school psychologist.

Teachers need to be alert to how children are responding to overall performance expectations. Most parents want their children to be successful, and sometimes expectations for performance cause unnecessary stress in children. In addition, teachers should pay specific attention to any unrealistic expectations or "irrational thinking" voiced by children about their own expectations for success. It is important to listen to the language that

TABLE 2.7. Major Characteristics, Educational Concerns and Complications, and Additional Resources for Students with Stress-Related Conditions

Major characteristics	Educational concerns and complications	Additional resources
• May be difficult to distinguish from symptoms of minor illness. • Irritability, nervousness, or inattentiveness • Difficulties adapting to change in routine • Clinginess • Use of key words such as *sad* or *afraid* • Attention-seeking behaviors • Mood changes • Isolation from peers • Posttraumatic stress disorder (PTSD), often related to specific event, typically results in increased nervousness and anxiety.	• Possible changes in quality of schoolwork. • Child may complain of headaches, stomachaches, or general body aches. • Child may become involved in fights or avoid classroom activities. • Pay specific attention to child's unrealistic expectations (e.g., perfectionism). • Rehearsal of stressful situations and relaxation techniques may be helpful.	• National Network for Child Care: *http://www.nncc.org* • The Educational Resources Information Center: *http://www.ericsp.org/pages/digests/PTSD.html* • New York University Child Study Center: *http://www.aboutourkids.org/articles/stress.html*

children use when they describe stressful events or situations. Listening well reassures them that the teacher is supportive of them, even as it gives the teacher some idea of what is going on in their daily lives.

One of the more useful ways we can assist children with stress reduction is to (1) teach them how to identify stress, (2) acknowledge that we all experience these stresses, and (3) describe specific coping skills for them. Rehearsal or role playing of stressful situations can sometimes be very fun as well as an effective stress-reduction tool. Relaxation techniques that combine visualization (i.e., thinking about pleasant things), breathing, and a cognitive strategy—for example, thinking the words "I'm okay now," "I'm going to get better," or "Things are under my control" while visualizing a favorite scene (e.g., the beach, a meadow, Mommy's lap) and breathing deeply and slowly—are useful strategies that can be taught to kids in the classroom to help them cope with stress. Table 2.7 summarizes the main characteristics, impact on education, and additional resources for dealing with students who have stress-related disorders.

Enuresis

Enuresis, otherwise known as bed-wetting or pants-wetting, is the involuntary releasing of urine into the bed or pants. Nocturnal enuresis, wetting the bed during sleeping hours, is more common in children than diurnal or daytime enuresis. Diurnal enuresis is more likely to effect the school environment. Enuresis is more prevalent in younger school-age children (15–20% of 5-year-olds), decreases significantly with age (7–10 % of 11-year-olds), and is rare (under 3%) by the age of 18. Males are nearly two times more likely to have problems with enuresis than females. Children from low socioeconomic backgrounds are at higher risk, and African American boys and girls are at higher risk, even when accounting for socioeconomic status. Although most children with enuresis do not have a psychiatric illness, psychological factors such as stress (e.g., family disruption, loss, or trauma) can play an important role in the onset of enuresis after a child has established periods of dryness. Enuresis can cause negative feelings in children, such as shame, embarrassment, anxiety, fear, and shyness or withdrawal, which may contribute to low self-esteem. Although enuresis normally decreases with time, treatments can speed up the process and help to prevent or minimize the negative psychological impact of wetting. Most parents and some school personnel try to help the child by limiting fluid intake and increasing opportunities to use the bathroom. However, these approaches have been shown to have minimal positive effect. Rather, treatments such as behavior modification programs and medications have been demonstrated to be more effective.

The most important impact that enuresis may have in the school setting involves negative social experiences. Enuresis can interfere with normal social activities, and children may become withdrawn and choose not to participate in important peer activities. Alternatively, children who wet their pants in the presence of other children may become the target of teasing, harassing, and peer exclusion. Such experiences can be humiliating for children, further increasing their feelings of shame, anxiety, and low self-esteem. (See Chapter 6 for more specific information on teasing and inclusion.) Behavioral treatments for enuresis will likely involve school personnel, especially if daytime wetting is targeted for

TABLE 2.8. Major Characteristics, Educational Concerns and Complications, and Additional Resources for Students with Enuresis

Major characteristics	Educational concerns and complications	Additional resources
• Involuntary wetting of bed or clothes • Improves with age • Feelings of shame • Embarrassment • Fear • Social isolation • Teasing • Low self-esteem	• Social isolation • Teasing • Must keep dry set of clothes for child. • Helpful to provide behavioral program in school.	• Health-Nexus: *http://www.health-nexus.com/enuresis-bed-wetting.htm* • Aetna InteliHealth: *http://www.intelihealth.com/IH/ihtIH/WSIHW000/9339/9898.html* • British United Provident Association: *http://hcd2.bupa.co.uk/fact_sheets/Mosby_factsheets/Nocturnal_Enuresis.html*

improvement. School personnel may also be asked to keep a clean change of clothes and to communicate regularly with parents regarding this problem. Table 2.8 summarizes the main characteristics, impact on education, and additional resources for dealing with students who have enuresis.

Gastrointestinal Disorders

There are many different gastrointestinal disorders; some of the more common ones in children include peptic ulcer, inflammatory bowel disease (including Crohn's disease and ulcerative colitis), and constipation/encopresis. Table 2.9 summarizes the main characteristics, impact on education, and additional resources for dealing with students who have gastrointestinal conditions.

Peptic Ulcer

Peptic ulcer is a recurring condition characterized by sores (ulcers) in the esophagus, stomach, or parts of the small intestines. Although in the past, ulcers were thought to be linked directly to stress responses, there is much more evidence now that certain organisms or diseases cause them. There is a lot of evidence that ulcer diseases occur in families, suggesting some kind of a genetic predisposition. There is also evidence that links smoking and certain medications to irritations of the stomach. There are few data to suggest that intake of particular foods and beverages causes ulcers.

The most common symptom of peptic ulcers is pain in the stomach or just above the middle of the chest. Most often, ulcers tend to negatively affect the person's willingness to eat appropriate amounts of nutritious food.

Effective treatment is aimed at controlling the peptic ulcer disease. Usually the first line of treatment is some form of antibiotics. Frequently, more state-of-the-art medications that "block" stomach acid secretion are used as well. These have been very successful in reducing ulcer problems and pain. The overall goals in the treatment of peptic ulcer are to

TABLE 2.9. Major Characteristics, Educational Concerns and Complications, and Additional Resources for Students with Gastrointestinal Conditions

Major characteristics	Educational concerns and complications	Additional resources
• Peptic ulcer • Pain in stomach or just above middle of chest • Certain foods may produce discomfort. • Inflammatory bowel disease (includes Crohn's disease and ulcerative colitis) • Weight loss • Diarrhea • Tenderness in abdomen • Blood in stool • Encopresis/stool soiling • Caused by constipation • Straining during bowel movements • Stomach pain • Bloating • Crankiness • Tiredness • Loss of appetite • Wetting • Reluctance to use the toilet	• Children may experience pain and discomfort in school. • Prearrange a plan for responding to difficulties in school. • Scheduled toilet sittings for children with encopresis may be necessary. • Be alert for crankiness and stomach pain associated with ongoing constipation.	• Penn State Children's Hospital: *http://www.hmc.psu.edu/ childrens/healthinfo/i/ibd.htm* • Crohn's amd Colitis Foundation of Canada: *http:// www.ccfc.ca/en/info/brochures/ parents.html* • KidsHealth: *http:// kidshealth.org/parent/medical/ digestive/peptic_ulcers_p2.html* • Keep Kids Healthy: *http:// www.keepkidshealthy.com/ welcome/conditions/ encopresis.html*

relieve the pain, heal the ulcer, and prolong the intervals between recurrences. The nonsurgical or medical treatment of ulcer disease is one of attempted control, not cure. Medications such as cimetidine (Tagamet), which decreases the acidity of stomach contents, are among the more widely used medicines. Compliance with the daily dosage is essential, however, if the medication is to have its maximal effect. Finally, there is little evidence that dietary intake causes peptic disease or that dietary therapy is useful as a form of treatment. This finding goes against a lot of historical medical and folk thinking. Nevertheless, people are generally encouraged to avoid foods that produce discomfort.

Inflammatory Bowel Disease

Inflammatory bowel disease refers to a group of illnesses that cause inflammation and/or ulceration in the lining of the bowel. The disease is often chronic and long term, with a very unpredictable outcome. Symptoms usually consist of weight loss, diarrhea, tenderness in the abdomen, and sometimes blood in the stool. Two of the most common conditions classified as inflammatory bowel disease are Crohn's disease and ulcerative colitis. Crohn's disease is often very difficult to treat, quite painful, and frequently characterized by lifelong exacerbations and recurrences. Whereas Crohn's disease occurs in the segments of the small intestine, ulcerative colitis affects the small bowel or the colon—the large intestine. The usual symptoms include cramp-like stomach pain and occasionally bloody diarrhea. Ulcerative colitis can be a serious and chronic problem, further compounded by malnutrition. Surgical intervention is often a treatment of choice.

These gastrointestinal disorders cause pain and discomfort in children, whether at home or in school. Consult the parents to ascertain the doctor's recommendations for optimal response and management during painful episodes. Pay special attention to the child's pallor and expression, ask questions about how he or she is feeling, and draw upon a prearranged plan containing the parents' as well as the doctor's suggestions for responding to these difficulties when they occur at school. Many of the suggestions in Chapter 6 are also helpful in this area as well.

Encopresis/Stool Soiling

Stool soiling affects about 2% of children. Most often, this type of soiling occurs because of constipation; however, in a very few children, it is caused by a disease or a birth defect. Stool soiling caused by constipation is called *encopresis*. In children with encopresis, there is usually some form of blockage in the lower bowel because of large stool and leakage soiling. It is important to remember that this type of stool soiling is involuntary—the child does not often mean to soil his or her pants. Soiling can occur occasionally or many times a day. Symptoms of constipation include extreme straining during a bowel movement, stomach pain, bloating, crankiness, fatigue, loss of appetite, wetting, and general reluctance to use the toilet. Constipation often occurs because of dietary limitations and lack of sufficient fluids. However, in many children constipation simply occurs periodically and cannot be explained. A tendency toward constipation runs in some families. Additionally, an illness that leads to poor food intake, physical inactivity, or fever can also result in constipation and stool soiling that remain as problems after the illness goes away.

After the doctor has determined that the child has some form of constipation, a general bowel training program is usually suggested and a stool softener recommended. Often the child has to spend a certain amount of time sitting on the toilet at scheduled intervals. Accomplishing these "seatings" requires cooperation among school personnel and a sensitive awareness of these issues. Teachers need to know if constipation remains an issue for a child so that they can consult with the family and doctor regarding the scheduled toileting program. It is important to remain alert for crankiness and obvious stomach pain associated with ongoing constipation.

Blood Disorders

There are many blood disorders that affect thousands of schoolchildren in the United States. Some of these disorders are very rare and some are more common. More common blood disorders include anemia (deficiency of oxygen-carrying capacity), sickle cell disease, hemophilia (inability to stop bleeding), and various cancers of the blood such as leukemia (see section on cancer). Symptoms depend on the specific disorder but may include lack of energy, recurrent infections, diarrhea, jaundice, excessive bleeding that does not

TABLE 2.10. Major Characteristics, Educational Concerns and Complications, and Additional Resources for Students with Blood Disorders

Major characteristics	Educational concerns and complications	Additional resources
• Lack of energy • Recurrent infections • Diarrhea • Jaundice • Excessive bleeding that does not stop • Swollen hands and feet • Pain • Irritability • Fever	• Emergency procedures must be in place for dealing with injuries or episodes of bleeding. • Children may be restricted from activities that may result in injury. • Children may need medication and close monitoring. • Cognitive deficits may result. • Expect frequent/unpredictable hospitalizations and school absences. • Special diets may be required.	• Keep Kids Healthy: *http://www.keepkidshealthy.com/welcome/commonproblems/anemia.html* • Sickle Cell Disease Association of America: *http://www.sicklecelldisease.org/what_is.htm* • Keep Kids Healthy: *http://www.keepkidshealthy.com/welcome/conditions/hemophilia.html* • American Cancer Society: *http://www.cancer.org/docroot/cri/cri_2_1x.asp?dt=24*

stop, swollen hands and feet, pain, irritability, and fever. These mostly genetic conditions can be associated with national heritage. For example, sickle cell anemia is associated with African American descent, whereas other forms of anemia are associated with Mediterranean descent. The most common cause of anemia in school-age children is a lack of iron in the diet. Treatments for blood disorders also depend on the specific disorder, but generally children must be seen regularly by their doctor, receive immunizations, and take medications.

Children with blood disorders are likely to need a special education plan to address the specific challenges within the school environment. For children with bleeding disorders, emergency procedures must be in place to deal with possible injuries or episodes of bleeding. These children are usually restricted in activity (e.g., they do not participate in physical education activities, where injury may occur). These children may need to be closely supervised and monitored during school hours. Cognitive deficits may result from the disorder itself or from the side effects of the treatments. Hospitalizations and school absences may be unpredictable, frequent, and for long periods of time. Special diets may be needed, which affect lunches, snack times, and special events such as birthday treats. Table 2.10 summarizes the main characteristics, impact on education, and additional resources for dealing with children who have blood disorders.

Migraine

Much like adults, children can experience headaches for many reasons. Some headaches are caused by stress, fever, or trauma to the head, and some have an unknown origin. For the most part headaches are a temporary, unpleasant problem that resolves in a short time and has little impact on the child's long-term school performance. However, some children have chronic, severe migraines that interfere with their ability to attend and benefit from school. Migraines are caused by dilation and constriction of the blood vessels in the brain. Migraines tend to run in families, and some forms are known to have specific triggers, such as bright or flashing lights, stress, or certain food products (e.g., chocolate or wine). There are several types of migraines, identified by the part of the brain involved and the resulting symptoms that children experience. For the most part, migraines are characterized by severe pain in a part of the head (e.g., behind one eye) or the whole head, extreme sensitivity to light and sound, dizziness, nausea, and vomiting. Other symptoms can include visual distortions, muscle weakness, and associated motor difficulties. Treatments for migraines typically are aimed at relieving symptoms and preventing future episodes. The effectiveness of medications varies widely, so some children benefit greatly, whereas others receive no benefit.

Frequent migraines can cause excessive absence and produce anticipatory anxiety in children. In addition, anxiety, depression, and behavioral problems may be associated. Children fearing the onset of a migraine may find it hard to concentrate on schoolwork. In

TABLE 2.11. Major Characteristics, Educational Concerns and Complications, and Additional Resources for Students with Migraines

Major characteristics	Educational concerns and complications	Additional resources

• Caused by blood vessels either constricting or narrowing or expanding or dilating
• Although head pain is usually on one or both sides of the head, a child may complain of feeling pain all over.
• Throbbing or pounding pain
• Sensitivity to light and sound
• May experience motor difficulties (e.g., stumbling or feeling uncoordinated).
• Abdominal discomfort
• Accompanied by nausea, decreased appetite, or vomiting.
• Children may appear pale in the face.
• Excessive sweating
• Aura (occasional feeling presaging a migraine)
  • See flashing lights or vision becomes blurred.
  • Feel as if they are smelling something odd.
	• Impacts vision.
	• Sudden onset and need to respond with medication require teacher flexibility in allowing the student to leave class or lie down to relax.
	• Can trigger irritability or depression, leading to behavior problems.
	• Fear of onset leads to difficulty in concentrating or feeling preoccupied.
	• Triggered by stress that may be associated with test anxiety, school performance, and social situations.
	• Leads to frequent school absences.
		• National Headache Foundation: http://www.headaches.org
		• National Headache Foundation: http://www.headaches.org/consumer/educationalmodules/childrensheadache/agmigrainevariants.html
		• The Cleveland Clinic: http://www.clevelandclinic.org/health/health-info/docs/2500/2555.asp?index=9637

many cases, the need to administer medication as early as possible necessitates that the teacher and child have a plan in place for immediate action upon the onset of a migraine. Table 2.11 summarizes the main characteristics, impact on education, and additional resources for dealing with children who have migraines.

Heart Conditions

According to the American Heart Association, congenital heart defects are the most common cardiovascular problems in children, with 8–10 children per 1,000 affected. Other cardiovascular conditions that affect children include heart murmurs and hypertension (high blood pressure). Most of the congenital heart problems are associated with other genetic conditions such as Down syndrome. Symptoms of such heart conditions may include fatigue, inability to exercise vigorously, colored patches in the skin, failure to thrive, delayed or stunted growth, racing or irregular pulse, labored breathing, and swelling of toes or fingers, giving a club-like appearance. Treatments range from surgical procedures to a wait-and-watch approach; many children fall in the middle of this range, requiring some medication and/or restricted activity. The outcome for children with such conditions varies greatly, depending on the type and severity of heart problem.

Depending on the severity, heart conditions can present significant challenges within the school environment. For children with mild conditions, a general awareness and minimal level of monitoring may suffice. In contrast, children with more severe heart problems may require much more attention. These children often need an IEP that incorporates

TABLE 2.12. Major Characteristics, Educational Concerns and Complications, and Additional Resources for Students with Heart Conditions

Major characteristics	Educational concerns and complications	Additional resources
• Fatigue • Labored breathing • Skin color irregularity • Swelling of toes or fingers • Stunted growth	• Because these students tire more quickly, they may look as if they are inattentive or slow learners. • Difficulty engaging in physical education or physically demanding activities. • Child may be anxious about condition and complications that could occur. • School personnel need to be trained in CPR. • Experience teasing due to physical appearance or limitations. • School day may be interrupted by attending to medication regimen.	• American Heart Association: *http://www.americanheart.org/ presenter.jhtml?identifier=1477* • Congenital Heart Information Network: *http://www.tchin.org/* • Heart Children New Zealand: *http:// www.heartchildren.org.nz/book/ hcbookindex.htm*

special educational and medical needs. It is essential for all relevant school personnel to be educated about the condition, its consequences, and their role in providing support. Information from the children's physician is essential to determine appropriate levels of exercise. Both children and school personnel may be anxious about the potential for cardiac failure. It is essential that the homeroom teacher, physical education instructor, and other appropriate personnel be trained in administering CPR. Children whose activities are limited or who show stunted growth or deformities may be teased and excluded by other children (see Chapter 6), which needs to be handled by school personnel. Cognitive deficits resulting from, or associated with, the heart conditions (e.g., Down syndrome) may require additional educational accommodations. Clear communication among health care providers, school personnel, the child, and his or her family is essential. Table 2.12 summarizes the main characteristics, impact on education, and additional resources for dealing with children who have heart conditions.

Infectious Diseases

Infectious diseases are conditions that may be passed from one child to the next through a spreading of viruses or bacteria. It is safe to say that all children will come in contact with, and become sick from, viruses and bacteria. Though many of these viruses and bacteria can create significant short-term problems (e.g., the influenza virus), in most cases children recover and return to school with little or no lingering effects of their illness. However, more severe illnesses and consequences are associated with such viruses as hepatitis and HIV as well as illnesses caused by bacteria such as bacterial meningitis. HIV has garnered the most press. Other infectious diseases include hepatitis A, B, and C, meningitis, polio, chickenpox, sexually transmitted diseases, mononucleosis, tuberculosis, and more recently, the West Nile virus. Here I focus on the more severe diseases that have a significant, chronic impact on a child in school.

Children with severe communicable diseases are a major challenge for the school, particularly the classroom teacher. In addition to the secondary effects of the conditions and their treatments, such as cognitive decline, school personnel must be vigilant in preventing the spread of such diseases in the school. Consequently, school personnel may need to be trained in special precautionary measures to ensure that the child is appropriately and safely integrated into the classroom. Additionally, parents of well children may become concerned about their child "getting" the infectious disease. Consequently, the issue of whom to tell, what to tell, and when to tell others is of major importance and can pose real ethical and legal dilemmas for school officials. (The issue of disclosure is discussed more in Chapter 5.) Because of their classmates' fears, children with infectious diseases may become isolated and teased by other children. The characteristics and impact of infectious diseases varies significantly, precluding detailed coverage here. Table 2.13 summarizes the main characteristics, impact on education, and additional resources for dealing with children who have infectious diseases such as hepatitis or HIV. Additional Web-based resources are listed that provide general information on infectious diseases.

TABLE 2.13. Major Characteristics, Educational Concerns and Complications, and Additional Resources for Students with Infectious Diseases

Major characteristics	Educational concerns and complications	Additional resources

• Hepatitis A
  • Jaundice
  • Fatigue
  • Abdominal pain
  • Loss of appetite
  • Nausea
  • Diarrhea
  • Fever
• Hepatitis B
  • Jaundice
  • Fatigue
  • Abdominal pain
  • Loss of appetite
  • Neausea, vomiting
  • Joint pain
• HIV/AIDS
  • Rapid weight loss
  • Dry cough
  • Recurring fever
  • Profound fatigue
  • Diarrhea
  • White spots or unusual blemishes on the tongue, in the mouth, or in the throat
  • Blotches on or under the skin
  • Memory loss, depression, or other neurological disorders
	• Hepatitis A
	  • Can be spread through feces in children's bathrooms.
	  • Can be spread from mouth to mouth.
	• Hepatitis B and HIV/AIDS
	  • Can be spread through feces in children's bathrooms.
	  • Can be spread through blood and bodily fluids.
	• Strict ethical restrictions protect confidentiality and student's condition.
	• Social isolation
	• Teasing
	• Excessive absences
	• Given the fluid requirements that some medications require, students should be given ample water and restroom breaks.
	• Deterioration of the central nervous system in HIV can lead to cognitive difficulties and decrease in academic performance.
	• School personnel should be trained in standard precautionary procedures in medical emergencies with these students.
		• Center for Disease Control: *http://www.cdc.gov/ncidod/hip/GUIDE/infect.htm*
		• American Academy of Pediatrics: *http://www.aap.org/policy/re9950.html*
		• Band-Aides and Blackboards: *http://www.faculty.fairfield.edu/fleitas/healthed.html*
		• Infection Spotlight: *http://www.infectionspotlight.com*
		• National Foundation for Infectious Diseases: *http://www.nfid.org/*

CONCLUDING COMMENTS

This chapter provides an overview of the most frequent medical conditions that are likely to affect children in school. For more detailed information, see *Health-Related Disorders in Children and Adolescents: A Guidebook to Understanding and Educating* (Phelps, 1998), which provides an excellent overview of 96 medical conditions found in children and adolescents. This book can serve as an excellent source of information on rare and unusual genetic and acquired medical conditions that may impact children in the school environment.

Although this chapter outlines the general characteristics and effects of medical conditions on children, I would add the caution that all children respond differently to illnesses and their treatments. This difference occurs at both a biological and social level: Children respond differently to the same medication, and some children will be less negatively affected in school due to effective coping skills and good social support. Generalizing symptoms of illnesses and their effects on children is helpful to understand and identify cases in which children need help, but it is always essential to examine each child's situation individually. Do not assume that what works for one child will work for another. Unique aspects of the child's illness, coping skills, home life, and unrelated needs are important determinants of whether an educational intervention is necessary or successful. Additional discussions of individualizing interventions appear in Chapters 4, 5, and 6.

3

Legal Responsibilities
of the School

CHAPTER OBJECTIVES

Schools have a legal obligation to provide appropriate education to children and adolescents with chronic illness and/or disabilities. Over time, federal legislation has evolved that provides specific guidelines to educators outlining the responsibilities and process by which schools are obligated to address educational issues with children who have an illness or disability. The purpose of this chapter is to provide (1) a historical background of how the need for such educational services has emerged, and (2) specific information regarding each of the federal legislative actions that directly influence the provision of educational services to students with a chronic illness. To avoid getting bogged down in the details of the laws, I focus on the general meaning and interpretation of the laws and highlight the specifics that are essential for educators to know. Specific objectives for this chapter are to:

- To review the history of chronic illness in the schools and the evolving need for special services
- To identify pertinent federal legislation that bears directly on the school's responsibility for education of students with an illness or disability
- To emphasize the main points of each of the major legislative actions
- To introduce the process by which schools fulfill their legal obligations

31

HISTORICAL OVERVIEW

The concept of providing special education services to children with chronic illness in mainstream schools is relatively new, due mainly to the fact that prior to advances in medical technology, most of these children died or were so severely affected that education was not even a consideration. However, over time the culture and attitudes toward disability has moved from one of isolationism to inclusion. Spencer, Fife, and Rabinovich (1995) provide an excellent overview of how these forces led to the need and demand for educational services, and eventually to the federal legislation mandating schools to provide such services. A summary of this overview is provided here, and you are encouraged to see the original reference for more details.

Prior to the Civil War, virtually no children with chronic illness attended schools. If they were lucky enough to survive, these children almost never received a formal education. Special schools were built for children with chronic illness after the Civil War, but the children were largely kept from public view. During this phase of history, poverty and a lack of significant numbers of surviving children limited the extent to which there was a need or available resources to deal with this issue. Those few who were able to attend school were faced with a system that made no allowances for their limitations; it is likely that they were dismissed, if they could not keep up with their peers.

Social changes that occurred in the early 1900s led to laws that mandated school attendance for all children, including those with an illness or disability. Despite the law requiring these students to attend, little or no accommodations were made for them. Rather, these children were often placed in special classes or schools for children with developmental delays, which served as the catch-all location for any children who were different. Additionally, concerns regarding polio and tuberculosis led to an even greater trend of segregation.

By the mid-1900s, increased survival rates after World War II led to more children with chronic illness seeking entrance into regular classrooms. Despite this period, schools were not equipped to handle such students and often excluded them from regular educational opportunities. Children with chronic illness continued to face discrimination, exclusion, and limited educational opportunities.

The issue of civil rights for all Americans was the foremost issue on the national political stage in the early 1970s. During this time parents of children with illness or disability were demanding fair and equal treatment of their children regarding education. In several instances, school systems were taken to court as parents made allegations of civil rights infringements on behalf of these children, who were subjected to exclusion, segregation, and denial of an adequate education. These pressures and lower court rulings led to the passing of the first federal legislation in 1975 mandating fair and equal educational opportunities for children with illness or disability. However, a few years prior to this law, federal legislation was passed to prohibit discrimination based on disability, and this ruling had important implications for educational services for children with chronic illness and disability.

THE REHABILITATION ACT OF 1973

The Rehabilitation Act of 1973 (Public Law 93-112) is an update of the previously passed Vocational Rehabilitation Act, and clearly delineates the rights of people with disabilities, guaranteeing equal opportunities in areas such as public access, transportation, employment, and government services. In the case of children with chronic illness, this law applies to opportunities in education as well. For example, adolescents with a chronic illness or disability are guaranteed fair and equal access to educational and vocational resources, and legal recourse is available if discrimination occurs. Whereas most of this law pertains to disability issues outside of education, a small portion of the law (Section 504) has come to represent the most important aspect for education. Section 504 states:

> No otherwise qualified handicapped individual . . . shall, solely by reason of his handicap, be excluded from the participation in, be denied the benefits of, or be subjected to discrimination under any program or activity receiving Federal financial assistance.

In essence, the law states that any entity receiving federal funds must not discriminate, which obviously includes schools. The outcome of this law led to the formation of the *504 plan*, which is a plan for educational accommodations. This plan falls under the responsibility of general educational programs. An educational plan can be drawn up that provides some accommodations without the placement of the child in special education and the full implementation of an IEP (described below). The specific advantages and disadvantages to utilizing a 504 plan versus an IEP are discussed in more detail in Chapter 4.

THE EDUCATION FOR ALL HANDICAPPED CHILDREN ACT OF 1975

The Education for All Handicapped Children Act of 1975 (EHA; Public Law 94-142) is perhaps the greatest piece of legislation thus far to address the educational needs of children with chronic illness, and it serves as the backbone of the rights of all children to a fair and equal education. Basic principles of this law are listed in Table 3.1. The law requires schools to work with parents of children with an illness or disability to develop an education plan to address each child's needs through provision of services in the school. This plan is known as the individualized education plan, or IEP, which remains the basis for provision of services to chronically ill children today. (The IEP is discussed in more detail in Chapter 4.)

For the first time schools were mandated to provide services to children that were formerly considered to be outside their responsibility. These services included adjusting the curriculum (e.g., workload, pace, presentation), administration of medication, provision of therapies (e.g., speech, occupational, physical), provision of transportation, and even tutor-

TABLE 3.1. Basic Principles of the Individuals with Disabilities Education Act

- Each child with a qualifying disability must be educated in the least restrictive environment.
- In most cases, each child with an illness or disability must have a written individualized education plan (IEP) if requested by the child's parents.
- Services necessary for each child to improve his or her education should be clearly outlined in the IEP.
- An IEP is good for 1 calendar year and can be continued, amended, or discontinued yearly.
- Parents of children have rights to due process with recourse for grievances through the state educational system or civil courts.

ing. This was a radical change for school personnel, who were inexperienced and ill-equipped to provide such comprehensive services to children with such a wide variety of illness and/or disabilities, resulting in wide-ranging needs.

Public Law 94-142 came into effect in 1978 for children between the ages of 6 and 17 years. In 1980 the age range for eligibility for services was increased to include children between the ages of 3 and 21 years, which substantially increased the number of children for which the schools were responsible. For children who qualified, services were now mandated under numerous categories (listed in Table 3.2). Specifically, the "Other Health Impaired" category included children with any form of chronic health condition, including cancer, diabetes, asthma, seizures, and so on. Most importantly, this legislation mandated that each child with a disability or chronic illness was guaranteed the right to the same educational opportunities as any other child, and the law provided a mechanism for legal recourse against the schools if these rights were violated.

Several amendments were made to Public Law 94-142 over the next decade or so, although modifications varied by state. In many states the age ranges were expanded so that children from birth to age 3 years were eligible for early intervention services (Public Law 99-457). Not only did this mean that more children would receive services, but it reflected a shift toward early intervention that had not been emphasized previously. Additionally, early developmental assessment was provided by school-based early intervention

TABLE 3.2. Students for Whom the Individuals with Disabilities Education Act Mandates Services If Needed

- Mentally challenged, mentally retarded, or cognitively impaired
- Deaf or hard of hearing
- Visually handicapped (impaired or blind)
- Speech impaired or delayed
- Learning disabled or impaired
- Physically or orthopedically handicapped or impaired
- Emotionally disturbed
- Autism
- Brain injured
- Otherwise health impaired (includes chronic illnesses such as asthma, cancer, diabetes, epilepsy, arthritis, etc.)

programs in cases where concerns of health care providers or parents resulted in requests for evaluation. I discuss additional changes to this law in more detail when I discuss the Individuals with Disabilities Education Act 1997 amendments. Additional information on the evaluation process is provided in Chapter 4.

THE INDIVIDUALS WITH DISABILITIES EDUCATION ACT

This expansion and revision of the original federal legislation was an important step because it continued to broaden the services available to students with chronic illness. The name of the original legislation (Education for all Handicapped Children Act) was changed to the Individuals with Disabilities Education Act (IDEA; Public Law 101-476). Mandated services were expanded to include assistive technology services as part of the IEP. This law also required the provision of transition services for adolescents to aid them in their passage into adulthood (e.g., educational and vocational services).

THE AMERICANS WITH DISABILITIES ACT OF 1990

The IDEA legislation has education as its primary focus, and its principles are formulated within an educational perspective. In contrast, the Americans with Disabilities Act (ADA; Public Law 101-336) has the issue of disability as its central theme and is an update of the Rehabilitation Act of 1973. In some ways, many of the issues for children with chronic illness are covered in the education-based legislation. This law is complementary in that it provides additional legal assurance for persons with disabilities. It should be noted that not all children with chronic illness qualify as disabled (discussed further in Chapter 4).

THE INDIVIDUALS WITH DISABILITIES
EDUCATION ACT AMENDMENTS OF 1997

In the early 1990s the Office of Special Education and Rehabilitation Services in the U.S. Department of Education was charged with evaluating the effectiveness of the IDEA since it was first enacted in 1975 (Public Law 94-142). A long and thorough process of evaluating the effects of the 1975 legislation included obtaining feedback from professional organizations, U.S. Department of Education officials, parent groups, and education officials. As a result of this process, Congress reauthorized the original IDEA legislation with some amendments, and the bill was signed into law by President Bill Clinton in June 1997. The U.S. Department of Education then published the final regulations for implementing the changes to the law in March of 1999. In general, these legislative changes resulted in a law that mandated greater rights for children with disabilities to receive educational services

TABLE 3.3. Summary of 1997 Amendments to IDEA Legislation

- Requirements for least restrictive environment are strengthened.
- Access to, and participation in, the general education curriculum for children with disabilities is emphasized.
- Rights of parents to be involved in decision making are strengthened.
- A positive, proactive approach to behavior problems is emphasized.
- Inclusion of children with disabilities in school reform efforts and state and districtwide assessments is emphasized.
- An outcome-based approach is made mandatory, meaning that the state must establish performance goals and indicators to measure progress.
- State and local agencies are encouraged to work together toward systemwide changes that link student progress with school improvement.

on an equal level to those of children without disabilities. Table 3.3 contains a summary of the most recent changes to the IDEA that were implemented in 1997 and 1999.

DRAWBACKS OF FEDERAL AND STATE LEGISLATION

Most people would agree that the legislation described above represents a huge step forward in mandating the civil rights of children with chronic illness or disability, and that clearly the result is that children will receive a much better education. However, these changes do not come without costs. Once this legislation was passed, schools were suddenly thrust into a domain that was traditionally outside the responsibility of educational institutions. The result was a huge increase in responsibility and cost to provide the substantial infrastructure that these services require—which, until then, did not exist, or barely existed, in schools.

The vaguest provision in these laws was that for "related services." In general, related services are associated with the illness or disability of the child, although they are often not directly related to education. Related services might include psychological counseling, provision of medical services (e.g., physical therapy, treatments such as insulin shots), storage and administration of medications, and transportation (see Table 3.4). Since many of these services are peripheral to educational instruction, many have argued that the cost to the schools is simply too great. In fact, in 1982 the Reagan administration tried unsuccessfully to relieve local school systems of responsibility for providing the related services outlined in Public Law 94-142, due to the cost and scope of the services. Research has revealed that many of the children who need related services are not getting them due to a lack of resources. Rather, the provision of services is based on what the school district has available, instead of what is actually needed by the students in that district (Walker, 1984). Table 3.5 lists some of the drawbacks of this legislation for schools.

In my experience, I have found that nearly all school personnel want what is best for all the children, including provision of services to which they are entitled. However, most personnel are also faced with the reality that the needs of the children in their school dis-

TABLE 3.4. Related School Services Needed by Schoolchildren with Chronic Illness

- Support therapies
    - Physical therapy
    - Occupational therapy
    - Speech and language therapy
- Schedule modifications
    - Shortened classes or school days
    - More frequent breaks
    - Longer time for getting from one place to another
- Modified physical education activities
- Transportation
    - To and from school
    - Between classes
- Building accessibility
- Toileting/lifting assistance
- Counseling services
    - School
    - Career
    - Mental health
    - Rehabilitation
- School health services
    - Administration of medications
    - Implementation of medical procedures or treatments
    - Emergency procedures

Note. From *Pediatric Clinics of North America, 31.* Walker, D. K. Care of chronically ill children in schools, 221–233. Copyright 1984 with permission from Elsevier.

TABLE 3.5. Drawbacks of Legislation for Schools

- Requires provision of services largely unrelated to classroom instruction.
- Substantial increase in costs
- Increased responsibility for larger infrastructure
    - Health facilities
    - Medical equipment
- Requires hiring more personnel from various professions
    - Physical, occupational, and speech therapists
    - Nurses
    - Psychologists/counselors
    - Physicians
    - Audiologists
- Increased legal liabilities
- Strain on resources results in downsizing or eliminating other educational services.

TABLE 3.6. Websites Containing More Information on Legislation

www.ideapractices.org/links/osers.php

This site, sponsored by the U.S. Department of Education, consists of numerous resources as part of the Special Education Technical Assistance and Dissemination Network. It contains many links and an excellent section on frequently asked questions with responses from experts.

www.wrightslaw.com

This is a commercial site that contains valuable information for parents, advocates, educators, and attorneys. The site contains up-to-date information about special education law and advocacy for children with disabilities.

www.ed.gov/about/offices/list/osers/index.html

The federal government site for the U.S. Department of Education Office of Special Education and Rehabilitation contains volumes of information on every aspect of special education legislation, including the *No Child Left Behind* legislation.

www.dredf.org/idea10.html

This website provides a good summary of the most recent changes in the IDEA legislation that were implemented in 1997.

---

trict greatly exceed the amount of available resources. Most often, the school lacks the necessary finances, resulting in a shortage of general personnel (e.g., classroom aides), specialized personnel (e.g., school nurses, counselors, health professionals), equipment, space, supplies, and training for personnel. Despite these limitations, it is essential for schools to find effective and efficient ways to provide the services mandated by federal law, both to maximally benefit the children and to minimize the school's legal liabilities.

CONCLUDING COMMENTS

The evolving recognition of the rights and educational opportunities for people who have disabilities has greatly benefited society. Table 3.6 contains a list of websites that provide more detailed information on the history and specifics of the pertinent legislation. It is critical in a society such as ours that children with chronic illness and disabilities are afforded opportunities to benefit from our educational system. Likewise, these opportunities have benefited nondisabled and non-ill children as well. For example, all children benefit from interactions with children who may be different in some important way. However, these mandates have not come without significant cost to the educational system. It is important to recognize that a limited number of resources exists for educational systems, so it is critical to find effective and efficient ways to provide the necessary accommodations that would allow the greatest number of children to be served. In the next chapter I focus on developing IEPs and 504 plans that address the individual needs of these children in the most efficient and effective manner, given the limited resources available to schools.

4

Making Accommodations

Developing 504 Plans
and Individual Education Plans (IEPs)

CHAPTER OBJECTIVES

As discussed in Chapter 3, schools have a legal obligation to provide appropriate services for children with chronic illness. In this chapter I examine in more detail the process by which school personnel, medical professionals, parents, and their children with chronic illness work together to develop a plan that addresses the children's unique needs. Topics explored include (1) the criteria for determining if an IEP or 504 plan is needed, (2) how children are referred, (3) the process of an evaluation, and (4) implementation of the evaluation results into an educational plan. The chapter concludes with three examples of 504 plans and IEPs to illustrate how assessment information is integrated into an educational plan for a child with chronic illness. Specific objectives of this chapter are:

- To review general characteristics of IEPs and 504 plans
- To identify the steps in developing an IEP or 504 plan
- To illustrate the development of IEPs and 504 plans for children with chronic illness through use of examples

WHAT IS A 504 PLAN
AND AN INDIVIDUAL EDUCATION PLAN?

504 Plan

As mentioned, the Rehabilitation Act of 1973 requires that school districts provide a free and appropriate education to children with a disability. A 504 plan is a formal, written educational plan designed to address the child's unique educational needs as a result of the disability. Any child who has a physical or mental impairment in a major life activity—seeing, hearing, speaking, breathing, walking, learning, working, caring for self, performing manual tasks—is eligible for services. Children with chronic illness are frequently affected in these areas and therefore qualify for services through a 504 plan. Most children with chronic illness can be well served by a 504 plan, without the need for an IEP. A child with a 504 plan is served through the regular educational program rather than the special education program. Children who do not qualify for special education under the Individuals with Disabilities Education Act (IDEA) may qualify for services through a 504 plan. Consequently, this service category is much broader and more inclusive than the categories listed under the IDEA. In fact, many parents prefer a 504 plan over an IEP because they perceive special education as a program for severely disabled or handicapped individuals, and they do not want their child to experience the stigma of placement in special education. A blank form of a 504 plan is provided as Worksheet 4.1 (p. 53).

Individual Education Plan

The IEP is a formal, written educational plan that is constructed for each student who qualifies under this legislation (see Table 3.2 in Chapter 3). The IDEA defines as eligible only students who have certain specified conditions, if conditions require specialized educational programming. The development and implementation of the IEP falls under the responsibility of the special education program within each school district. The IEP is typically much more detailed and comprehensive than the 504 plan, although this is not necessarily the case. Worksheet 4.2 (p. 54) is an example of an IEP form that outlines educational accommodations that are much more detailed and specific than those on the 504 plan form. In general, the IEP must be developed so that the child is educated in the least restrictive environment. Additionally, the IEP must be reviewed at the end of 1 calendar year; at that time it can be continued as is, amended, or discontinued.

Accommodations

The educational needs of children with chronic illness vary greatly, depending on their abilities independent of the illness, the type and severity of illness or condition, and their ability to cope with the associated learning, emotional, and social problems. Consequently, accommodations can range from minor ones, such as providing more time to get from one class to the next or sitting nearer the blackboard, to more significant ones, such as providing home visits, reducing workload, providing transportation, and carrying out medical procedures or treatments in school. Although IEPs are only required to be reviewed yearly, it may be necessary to review them more frequently, given that some illnesses may go into remission or flare up unexpectedly. Likewise, the impact an illness or its treatment has on the child can vary depending on timing and type of treatments. For example, a child with cancer is more likely to be adversely affected during chemotherapy and radiation treatments than during the periods between treatments. It is important for parents, school officials, and medical professionals to communicate clearly regarding the child's condition, treatment, and resulting school-related needs. Worksheet 4.3 (p. 56) contains an accommodations checklist for 504 plans. Although this list is not exhaustive, it provides a reference for identifying potential accommodations for both 504 plans and IEPs.

"When Do I Use a 504 Plan, and When Do I Need an Individual Education Plan?"

Parents and educators addressing the needs of children with chronic illness commonly ask: "When do I use a 504 plan, and when do I need an IEP?" Children with a chronic illness may qualify for a 504 plan if their illness interferes with a major life activity, yet they may not need, or qualify for, special education services and an IEP. For example, a girl with juvenile rheumatoid arthritis may be limited in one major life activity (e.g., running, walking) and will need accommodation in that area (e.g., more time to get from one class to another and an alternative activity during physical education class). However, she does not need a specifically designed instructional program or services. In many cases, particularly when the illness is not severe, a 504 plan is an adequate and desirable approach to meeting educational needs.

There are times, however, when special education services are necessary because of the illness's significant impact on the child's ability to attend and benefit from public education. These children typically qualify for special education services under the "Other Health Impaired" (OHI) category listed in the IDEA legislation. In such cases, an IEP is needed to fully address the significant and multiple needs of the child. For example, a girl with more severe rheumatoid arthritis may have needs that necessitate an IEP. She may be unable to write because of joint pain in her hands, she may be unable to walk, she may

TABLE 4.1. Level of Functioning and Program Modifications Associated with Severity of Impairment

	Level 1: Mild	Level 2: Mild to moderate	Level 3: Moderate	Level 4: Severe
Is the child handicapped?	No	Possibly	Yes	Yes
How does it affect the child's functioning?	Health impairment does not interfere with day-to-day functioning and learning.	Health impairment does not interfere with learning, but there is a possibility of unusual episodes or crises.	Health impairment either presents frequent crises or so limits the child's opportunity to participate in activities that learning is interrupted.	Health impairment is so severe that special medical attention is regularly needed. The child's opportunity for activity is so limited that he or she may not be able to participate in a regular classroom.

From *Pediatric Clinics of North America, 31*, 221–233. Walker, D. K. Care of chronically ill children in schools. Copyright 1984 with permission from Elsevier.

have intermittent and extended absences during disease flare-ups, she may be too fatigued to attend the whole school day, and she may need treatment during school hours (e.g., physical therapy, medications, counseling). In this case, an IEP is needed to address the numerous negative effects that the arthritis has on her ability to participate in educational programming. (Table 4.1 summarizes the modifications necessary, based on the child's level of impairment.)

PROCESS FOR OBTAINING A 504 PLAN OR AN INDIVIDUAL EDUCATION PLAN

The process of identifying a child who needs accommodations, conducting an assessment, and developing and implementing an educational plan can take months. Consequently, when there are questions or concerns that arise, it is best to start the process very early rather than waiting until the child exhibits a pattern of problems. Each step in the process is reviewed below.

Referral

Before children can receive accommodations, they must be identified as students who have a disability or illness that significantly interferes with a major life activity or with school functioning. Referrals are typically made by parents or school personnel. Usually a parent initiates contact with the school to notify the teacher of a child's illness or disability. However, some parents believe that disclosing the child's condition to school officials will have a negative impact on the child, so they choose not to do so. I believe that it is best for parents to communicate openly with school officials about their child's illness (discussed in more detail in Chapter 5). Children may also be identified by teachers who observe them struggling in school as a result of the illness. Sometimes parents request that medical professionals send a letter to the school describing the current medical condition and requesting school services for the child.

Once the child is identified, a verbal or written request can be made for a special education evaluation; it is recommended that parents request the evaluation in writing. Once the request is made, the school is required by law to conduct an evaluation within 60 days. The cost of the evaluation is the responsibility of the school; the parents are not obligated to pay for this assessment. In some cases, parents may request an independent evaluation by a pediatric psychologist or pediatric neuropsychologist, who specializes in assessment and treatment of pediatric illness. The cost of this independent evaluation is typically covered by the parents.

Evaluation

A multidisciplinary team conducts an evaluation to determine if the child's illness interferes with school. The evaluation includes assessment of the child's current health, learning abilities and achievement, speech and language, hearing, vision, social skills, physical abilities, and emotional–behavioral status. Table 4.2 lists the many sources of information collected as part of the evaluation. The evaluation must be sufficient to accurately assess the nature and extent of the illness or disability, its effect on major life activities, and the services needed and available. The team conducting the evaluation may include teachers, school psychologists, school counselors, audiologists, speech pathologists, occupational and physical therapists, and school nurses. If the child's health problems interfere with school, most likely the child will qualify for services under the OHI category. Some states use different terminology, referring to this category as the "Physically or Otherwise Health Impaired" (POHI).

It is important to collect information from other health care providers as well. In many cases, the physician or nurse will write a letter to the school or the parent outlining the severity of the illness, its impact on the child, and any accommodations deemed necessary for the child. It is a good idea to speak directly with the child's physician or nurse to obtain accurate and complete information. The physician–nurse team is an extremely valuable resource that should be utilized whenever possible. A pediatric psychologist may also provide input in the form of an independent evaluation and report or through contributions to the physician's letter. Information from the medical team can be critical, especially in cases where the illness is rare or particularly severe. Although the medical team is free to make recommendations regarding accommodations, it is the school officials in conjunction with the parents who make the final decisions regarding accommodations and services provided to the child. This decision point can be a time of contention (I discuss this phase further in Chapter 5, when I deal with issues of communication).

Team Conference

Once all the evaluation data are collected, the multidisciplinary team meets to go over the information. Parents typically attend this meeting to serve as advocates for their child and to provide a context for interpreting their child's behavior. The child may or may not attend the meeting; as a general rule, it is better to include the child if he or she is old

---

TABLE 4.2. Sources of Information for Evaluations

- Teacher observations
- School records (e.g., grades, attendance, disciplinary records, standardized test scores)
- Test results (e.g., IQ, achievement, motor skills, psychological)
- Child interview
- Parent interview
- Teacher interview
- Medical professional interview
- Medical records and medical team correspondence
- Child self-report rating scales
- Teacher rating scales
- Parent rating scales
- Daily work samples

---

enough to understand what is happening. Often a school administrator is also in attendance. The law requires that placement decisions be made by a group of persons knowledgeable about the child, the disability or illness, the meaning of the evaluation data, and placement options. Parents can also request the presence of an outside professional (e.g., pediatric psychologist, nurse) to help interpret the data, provide suggestions for accommodations, and serve as an advocate for the child. I have attended several meetings in that role, and parents have reported that it was very helpful. During this meeting a determination is made as to whether the student has a disability or illness, whether it interferes with a major life activity, whether accommodations will be necessary, and how to implement the accommodations, if needed, into an educational plan.

Once a determination is made that a child will need accommodations, the next decision concerns whether a 504 plan or an IEP would be most appropriate. As mentioned, this choice is determined by the nature of the services needed by the child and whether they can be provided through regular educational programming (504 plan); if they cannot, then special education services (i.e., IEP) are needed. In many cases, the 504 plan or the IEP is developed in this same meeting. It is often during this meeting that conflict arises due to parents' requests for services that exceed what a school can afford to support. Parents have the right to disagree with the outcome of the evaluation and/or the services offered by the school, if they believe the best interests of their child will not be served. In cases when the issues cannot be resolved among parents and school officials, the parents can pursue the issue through the State Board of Education or through the civil courts. I believe that how the parents and school personnel manage this pivotal meeting will largely influence the outcome of the educational programming. The educational plan (504 plan or IEP) must document clearly the nature of services provided. Table 4.3 lists the information that must be included in an IEP.

Implementation and Monitoring

It is important to implement the educational plan as soon as possible, especially since the child has likely been experiencing the negative school-related consequences of his or her illness or disability for quite some time. In an attempt to limit use of school resources, sometimes school officials suggest waiting until the beginning of the next term (e.g., tri-

---

TABLE 4.3. Required Information in the Individual Education Plan

- Assessment of the child's current level of educational performance
- Annual goals of the IEP
- Measurable objectives to meet the goals
- Services to be provided
    Type of service (e.g., transportation, counseling, physical therapy)
    Duration of service (e.g., start date and length of service)
    Service provider (e.g., school nurse, counselor, teacher)
- Time in special education classes and regular education classes
- Method of evaluation, including review of the IEP annually

---

mester, semester, or school year) to implement the plan. Both parents and educators should strive for implementing the plan as early as is feasible. Depending on the types of accommodations and services required, it may take some time to implement the plan. For example, teachers may have to be informed so that they can make curriculum modifications, school personnel may have to be trained to supervise or participate in treatments or illness management (i.e., administering medications, providing emergency services), and specialized transportation or educational equipment may have to be obtained.

Monitoring the impact of the services is essential. It is recommended that the 504 plan or IEP stipulate some method of regular (weekly or monthly) communication between the parents and the school regarding the child's performance in areas identified as needing services. Additionally, the parents or physician should notify the school if the illness or disability status of the child changes significantly. Establishing these communication guidelines fosters a collaborative approach that likely prevents problems from intensifying too severely before they are noticed and addressed. As noted, a review must be conducted each year to evaluate the child's progress and determine the effects of the accommodations and services. At the annual review meeting, one of four determinations can be made: services may be increased, maintained at current levels, decreased, or discontinued. A new evaluation must be conducted at least once every 3 years, and more frequently, if necessary.

CASE EXAMPLES

Here I describe case examples to illustrate the kinds of issues involved with various chronic illnesses and how accommodations can be implemented through 504 plans or IEPs.

Case Example 1: Diabetes 504 Plan

Carol is an 8-year-old second grader with diabetes. Her diabetes is under relatively good control, for the most part, although some problems have arisen lately that have raised concern with her parents. Specifically, Carol has been reprimanded in school by her teacher for "excessive" requests to go to the bathroom and for eating during classes. Carol has come home crying three times in the last week, stating that she does not want to go back to school. Her parents are upset because they believe that she is being reprimanded in school for taking appropriate responsibility for her diabetes. Carol's parents had met with her first-grade teacher the prior year to discuss her diabetes, and the result was a relatively trouble-free year. They made the assumption that Carol's second-grade teacher is aware of her condition, understands its impact on Carol in school, and has developed a plan for dealing with the issues associated with the diabetes. To deal with these latest problems, Carol's parents requested a referral for an educational assessment and plan.

An evaluation was conducted that revealed that Carol's academic performance in her classes has been good. Her teacher has recorded some concerns about "not following rules" and "disruptive classroom behaviors," but the teacher does not feel as though these behaviors have warranted action to this point. Assessment also revealed that Carol has a moderate level of anxiety about the possibility of feeling embarrassed in front of other children and fear of getting in trouble with the teacher. Her diabetes continues to be under relatively good control.

A team meeting with Carol's teacher, the principal, school nurse, and her parents was held to discuss the evaluation and school programming. Carol's teacher was unaware of the diabetes and consequently the need for special treatment of Carol. The team decided that a few accommodations, through the implementation of a 504 plan, would adequately address Carol's issues. Figure 4.1 contains the 504 plan accommodations designated for Carol. In an ideal world, Carol's parents would have met with her second-grade teacher prior to the start of the school year to discuss their daughter's condition, what special needs the teacher might expect Carol to have, and to create and agree on a plan that would address those issues.

Case Example 2: Asthma 504 Plan

Jim is a 12-year-old sixth grader who has had moderately severe asthma since early childhood. Since he will be attending a new school (middle school) this year, his parents requested to meet with his teacher prior to the school year to discuss his condition. Jim's parents brought with them to the meeting a copy of his 504 plan from fifth grade, a letter from his physician, and a notebook with a diary of his asthma condition and treatments. The teacher was very appreciative of the parents' efforts and scheduled a meeting with the 504 plan coordinator, the parents, a school administrator, and the teacher.

An abbreviated evaluation revealed that Jim had done well on his elementary school 504 plan. Concerns regarding triggers for his asthma, school activities, and his treatments were discussed. In the event that exposure to chemicals (science class) or other irritants (dust, pollen, smoke) would be likely, alternative activities and assignments were selected. Emergency protocols were discussed in the case of an asthma attack. Treatments were discussed and plans made for Jim to carry his inhaler at appropriate times. Figure 4.2 contains the 504 plan accommodations made for Jim. This scenario represents the optimal situation: Parents and school personnel work together to create an appropriate plan to prevent problems and to deal with problems *before* they actually occur.

Case Example 3: Juvenile Rheumatoid Arthritis 504 Plan

McKenzie is a 16-year-old high school junior with juvenile rheumatoid arthritis (JRA). She was diagnosed as a small child; the disease has largely stabilized, with only occasional flare-ups, during which time she can be severely but temporarily affected. She may miss 2 or 3 days of classes during these flare-ups, and she can have significant joint pain, swelling, and limited mobility for a week or two afterward. Because McKenzie has had JRA for several years, she is aware of the accommodations she needs to deal with its impact on her in the school setting. She requested a meeting be held with her parents, a 504 plan coordinator, and her homeroom teacher. During this meeting McKenzie asked for several accom-

School District: Any Community School District

Address: 123 W. Education Ave.

Any City, IA 01234

Student: Carol Hauser   **School:** Emmit Elementary   **Grade:** 2

Date of implementation: 11/24/02   **Review:** Annually

Statement of student's disability as it relates to this plan: Carol has diabetes that interferes with her self-care and learning.

Accommodation/strategy	Implementor(s)	Monitoring dates	Comments
Permission to get drinks and use restroom as needed	Teacher: Ms. Cole	Beginning of each month	No need to ask permission
Meet with school counselor weekly	Counselor: Mr. James	Monthly	Meet as needed
Snack as needed	Ms. Cole	Each semester	If snacking is disruptive, can go to nurse's office
Monitor insulin injections	School nurse	Monthly	Continue process in place since last year

cc. Parents/Guardians
Section 504 Coordinator
Educational Record
Principal
Teacher(s)

FIGURE 4.1. Completed Section 504 accommodations plan form for Carol Hauser.

47

School District: _Any Community School District_

Address: _123 W. Education Ave._

Any City, IA 01234

Student: _Jim Dandy_ **School:** _Tyler Middle School_ **Grade:** _6_

Date of implementation: _8/27/02_ **Review:** _Annually_

Statement of student's disability as it relates to this plan: _Jim has asthma that causes significant problems breathing. Asthma attacks may require emergency intervention._

Accommodation/strategy	Implementor(s)	Monitoring dates	Comments
Alternate science assignment	Teacher: Mr. Pancah	Monthly	As necessary
Use of library during recess	Librarian: Ms. Torrance	Monthly	When parents or Jim request (e.g., during high pollen counts)
Jim carries inhaler during Physical Education	Phys. Ed Teacher: Mr. Lewis	Monthly	
Can leave class to get inhaler from nurse	Nurse: Mr. Pancah	Monthly	No permission required
Teachers current in CPR	Principal Howard	Annually	All Jim's teachers current in CPR certification
Report asthma attacks	Principal Howard	Annually	Immediately report to school nurse, parents, principal.

cc: Parents/Guardians
Section 504 Coordinator
Educational Record
Principal
Teacher(s)

FIGURE 4.2. Completed Section 504 accommodations plan form for Jim Dandy.

48

modations at the time of her flare-ups. A brief review of McKenzie's records indicated that she has had a 504 plan for several years, from which has evolved several accommodations to address her problems. All that was necessary at this point was to request and discuss the accommodations, then document them after consensus was reached. Figure 4.3 contains the 504 plan accommodations for McKenzie. In this case, given McKenzie's age and maturity, she took the responsibility for requesting the 504 plan and asserting her needs in relation to her condition.

Case Example 4: Cystic Fibrosis IEP

Terrance is a 14-year-old seventh grader with cystic fibrosis (CF). Because of the severity of his condition, he is an unusually small and skinny child. He is frequently absent from school and is unable to stay in school the whole day when he does attend, due to fatigue. He is well below grade level in many of his courses due to his excessive absences and cognitive difficulties resulting from the CF and the medications. He is socially delayed for the same reasons and has few friends. Terrance is often teased at school, especially about being small and "wimpy."

Terrance's parents have requested an evaluation to determine his service needs in school at the beginning of each of his school years. Results of this current evaluation are consistent with previous evaluations: He is significantly below grade level in math, socially isolated, significantly anxious and depressed, extremely fatigued, and has numerous and sometimes extended absences. During the team meeting it was determined that Terrance has many needs, including remedial math, counseling, social skills training, percussive treatments, and medication administration during the school day, reduced workload, access to a teacher and books during absences, and a special diet. The team discussion resulted in a decision that special education services were needed.

Figure 4.4 contains the outline of an IEP for Terrance. Accommodations include time in remedial math class, home visits by a teacher during his absences, percussive treatments during class, alternative physical education requirements, reduced school days and a reduced workload, and a special diet. The IEP meeting was conducted with Terrance's input regarding the accommodations. The school nurse, principal, IEP coordinator, homeroom teacher, and Terrance's parents worked together to develop the IEP in Figure 4.4. In this case, Terrance's needs are clearly greater than what could be appropriately addressed with a 504 plan. Given his needs for remedial work, teacher visits to the home, special medical accommodations, and curricular modifications, it was necessary to enlist the resources of the special education department.

CONCLUDING COMMENTS

Many parents, educational professionals, and health care providers are confused and/or misinformed about 504 plans and IEPs. Their purpose is to best serve the child with a disability or health condition by ensuring a federally mandated, fair, and timely process of

School District: Any Community School District

Address: 123 W. Education Ave.

Any City, IA 01234

Student: McKenzie Wellington   **School:** West High School   **Grade:** 11

Date of implementation: 8/29/02   **Review:** Annually

Statement of student's disability as it relates to this plan: McKenzie has JRA that temporarily flares up, causing pain, swelling, and limited mobility. She may miss a few days of school during this time.

Accommodation/strategy	Implementor(s)	Monitoring dates	Comments
Teachers send work home if misses two or more days	Teachers	Annually	Send work home with Tammy—McKenzie's sister
Reduced assignments as necessary	Teachers	Annually	
Untimed exams/oral exams	Teachers	Annually	If finger pain or swelling
Excused tardiness to classes	Teachers	Annually	If difficulty walking

cc. Parents/Guardians
Section 504 Coordinator
Educational Record
Principal
Teacher(s)

FIGURE 4.3. Completed Section 504 accommodations plan form for McKenzie Wellington.

Special Education Services

Indicate the services, activities, and supports that will be provided in order for this individual: 1) to advance towards attaining the IEP goals; 2) to be involved and progress in the general curriculum; 3) by age 14, to pursue the course of study and post-high school outcomes (living, lifelong learning, and work); 4) to participate in extracurricular and other nonacademic activities; and 5) to be educated and participate with other individuals with disabilities and nondisabled individuals.

Y N Accommodations   Y N Linkages/interagency   Y N Supplementary aids and services
                                           responsibilites

Y N Assistive technology   Y N Program modifications   Y N Supports for school personnel

Y N Community experience   Y N Specially designed instruction   Y N Support or related services

Y N Development of work and other post-high school living objectives   Y N Other: _____

Describe each service, activity, and support indicated above:	Provider(s) and when the service, activity, or support will occur	Setting
1 hr. remedial math daily	Provider(s): Mr. Jones Time and frequency/when provided: 1hr. daily	_____ General education _X_ Special education _____ Community
Home visits	Provider(s): Ms. Jones Time and frequency/when provided: As needed	_____ General education _X_ Special education _____ Community
Course load reductions and activity modifications	Provider(s): All teachers Time and frequency/when provided: As necessary	_X_ General education _____ Special education _____ Community
Medical treatments as outlined in letter from physician	Provider(s): School Time and frequency/when provided: Daily as needed	_X_ General education _____ Special education _____ Community
Dietary restrictions—see file in nurse's office	Provider(s): All personnel Time and frequency/when provided: All times	_X_ General education _____ Special education _____ Community
	Provider(s): Time and frequency/when provided:	_____ General education _____ Special education _____ Community
	Provider(s): Time and frequency/when provided:	_____ General education _____ Special education _____ Community
	Provider(s): Time and frequency/when provided:	_____ General education _____ Special education _____ Community
	Total time removed from general education:	

FIGURE 4.4. Completed IEP outline for Terrance Striker.

TABLE 4.4. Websites Containing Information on Individual Education Plans and 504 Plans

www.familyvillage.wisc.edu/school.htm

This is the best website I found for information on 504 plans and IEPs. It is housed at the University of Wisconsin and contains dozens of links to all aspects of special education services for children with disabilities.

www.ed.gov/about/offices/list/osers/index.html

The U.S. Department of Education website contains a great deal of information on 504 plans and IEPs.

www.diabetes.org/main/community/advocacy/504plan.jsp

This site is hosted by the American Diabetes Association and contains sample 504 plans for children with diabetes. The information is also very useful for 504 plans and IEPs for other health problems as well.

www.chtu.org/504.html

This is the website of the Cleveland Heights Teachers Union. It contains an excellent section on frequently asked questions about 504 plans and other special education programming.

www.ldonline.org/ld_indepth/iep/iep_process.html

The Virginia Department of Education has created an excellent site that contains a great deal of information about developing IEPs in language that is easy to understand and access.

assessment and educational planning. Despite the federal mandate, many children fail to receive appropriate educational accommodations due to a shortage of resources in schools and inadequate advocacy on behalf of the child. Table 4.4 lists websites that provide more detailed information on 504 plans and IEPs, including frequently asked questions, sample plans for children with chronic illness, and suggestions for improving the quality of the process of planning and documenting accommodations.

WORKSHEET 4.1. Blank Section 504 Accommodations Plan Form

School District: _____

Address: _____

Student: _____ School: _____ Grade: _____

Date of implementation: _____ Review: _____

Statement of student's disability as it relates to this plan:

_____

_____

Accommodation/strategy	Implementor(s)	Monitoring dates	Comments

cc. Parents/Guardians
Section 504 Coordinator
Educational Record
Principal
Teacher(s)

WORKSHEET 4.2. Blank IEP Form

Name: _____ Date: ___ / ___ / ___ Page ___ of ___

Special Education Services

Indicate the services, activities, and supports that will be provided in order for this individual: 1) to advance towards attaining the IEP goals; 2) to be involved and progress in the general curriculum; 3) by age 14, to pursue the course of study and post-high school outcomes (living, lifelong learning, and work); 4) to participate in extracurricular and other nonacademic activities; and 5) to be educated and participate with other individuals with disabilities and nondisabled individuals.

Y N Accommodations   Y N Linkages/interagency responsibilites   Y N Supplementary aids and services

Y N Assistive technology   Y N Program modifications   Y N Supports for school personnel

Y N Community experience   Y N Specially designed instruction   Y N Support or related services

Y N Development of work and other post-high school living objectives   Y N Other: _____

Describe each service, activity, and support indicated above:	Provider(s) and when the service, activity, or support will occur	Setting
	Provider(s): Time and frequency/when provided:	____ General education ____ Special education ____ Community
	Provider(s): Time and frequency/when provided:	____ General education ____ Special education ____ Community
	Provider(s): Time and frequency/when provided:	____ General education ____ Special education ____ Community
	Provider(s): Time and frequency/when provided:	____ General education ____ Special education ____ Community
	Provider(s): Time and frequency/when provided:	____ General education ____ Special education ____ Community
	Provider(s): Time and frequency/when provided:	____ General education ____ Special education ____ Community
	Provider(s): Time and frequency/when provided:	____ General education ____ Special education ____ Community
	Provider(s): Time and frequency/when provided:	____ General education ____ Special education ____ Community
	Total time removed from general education:	

(continued)

Blank IEP Form *(page 2 of 2)*

Name: _____ Date: ___ / ___ / ___ Page ___ of ___

Special Education Services, continued

[ ] Yes   [ ] No   Are extended school year (ESY) services required? If yes, specify the goals that require ESY services and describe the services. _____

_____

[ ] Yes   [ ] No   Are specialized transportation services required that are related to the disability? If yes, describe.
   [ ] Special route (outside normal attendance area or transportation not typically provided based on distance from school)
   [ ] Attendant services   [ ] Specially equipped vehicle   [ ] Other _____

Physical Education: [ ] General [ ] Modified—describe below   [ ] Specially designed—requires goal(s)

_____

_____

Indicate how this individual will participate in districtwide assessments
   [ ] Without modifications or accommodations   [ ] With modifications or accommodations (describe below)
   [ ] Through the state alternate assessment

_____

_____

_____

Least Restrictive Environment Considerations

Address the following questions.

[ ] Yes   [ ] No   Will this individual receive all special education services in general education environments?
If no, explain: _____

_____

_____

[ ] Yes   [ ] No   Will this individual participate in nonacademic activities with nondisabled peers and have the same opportunity to participate in extracurricular activities as nondisabled peers?
If no, explain: _____

_____

_____

[ ] Yes   [ ] No   Will this individual attend the school he or she would attend if nondisabled?
If no, explain: _____

_____

_____

[ ] Yes   [ ] No   Will this individual attend a special school? If yes, attach responses to the special school questions.

Progress Reports

Parents: You will be informed of your child's IEP progress _____ times per year. You will receive:
[ ] An IEP report with cards and progress reports   [ ] Updated copies of the IEP goal pages
[ ] _____

WORKSHEET 4.3. Accommodation/Modification Checklist

Name: _____ Date: _____

Date form completed: _____ Form completed by: _____

Which of the following accommodations/modifications does the student need to be successful in the classroom?

PHYSICAL ARRANGEMENT OF ROOM/ENVIRONMENT

_____ Seating student near teacher

_____ Seating student near a positive role model

_____ Standing near the student when giving directions or presenting lessons

_____ Avoiding distracting stimuli (e.g., sounds of air conditioner, high traffic area, etc.)

_____ Increasing distance between desks

_____ Providing preferential seating

_____ Providing opportunity for movement

_____ Allowing use of headphones to block out distractions

_____ Altering physical arrangement of room

_____ Reducing/minimizing distractions (e.g., visual, auditory, spatial)

_____ Seating student near positive role model

_____ Offering cooling-off period/place

_____ Allowing alternate setting/mode for speeches/presentations

_____ *Additional accommodations:* _____

LESSON PRESENTATION

_____ Pairing students to check work

_____ Writing key points on the board

_____ Providing peer tutoring

_____ Providing visual aids, large print, films, organizational outlines

_____ Providing peer note taker

_____ Making sure directions are understood

_____ Including a variety of activities during each lesson

_____ Repeating directions to the student after they have been given to the class; then have him or her repeat and explain directions to teacher

_____ Providing written outline, listing key points and concepts˙

_____ Providing study guides

_____ Allowing for frequent conferences with instructor to check for understanding

_____ Allowing student to tape record lessons

_____ Having child review key points orally

_____ Teaching through multisensory modes (i.e., visual, auditory, kinestetics, olfactory)

(continued)

_____ Using computer-assisted instruction

_____ Providing a model or demonstration to help students; posting the model and referring to it often

_____ Accompanying oral directions with written directions for student reference

_____ Providing cross-age peer tutoring to assist the student in finding the main idea

_____ Underlining, highlighting, using cue cards, etc.

_____ Breaking longer presentations into shorter segments

_____ *Additional accommodations:* _____

ASSIGNMENTS/WORKSHEETS

_____ Allowing extra time to complete tasks

_____ Simplifying complex directions

_____ Handing worksheets out one at a time

_____ Highlighting key concepts on handouts

_____ Reducing the reading level of the assignments

_____ Requiring fewer correct responses to achieve grade (i.e., quality vs. quantity)

_____ Allowing student to tape record assignments/homework

_____ Providing a structured routine in written form

_____ Providing study skills training/learning strategies

_____ Giving frequent short quizzes and avoiding long tests

_____ Shortening assignments; breaking work into smaller segments

_____ Allowing typewritten or computer-printed assignments prepared by the student or dictated by the student and recorded by someone else, if needed

_____ Using self-monitoring devices

_____ Reducing homework assignments

_____ Not grading handwriting

_____ Not requiring cursive or manuscript writing

_____ Reversals or transpositions of letters and numbers should not be marked wrong, but pointed out for correction

_____ Not requiring lengthy outside reading assignments

_____ Monitoring by teacher of student's self-paced assignments (e.g., daily, weekly, biweekly)

_____ Arranging for homework assignments to reach home with clear, concise directions

_____ Recognizing and giving credit for student's oral participation in class

_____ Modifying expectations for assignments requiring speed and accuracy

_____ Providing alternative options for assignments

_____ Providing extra options for assignments

_____ *Additional accommodations:* _____

(continued)

TEXTBOOKS/MATERIALS

_____ Providing tape-recorded books and/or modified textbooks (e.g., lower reading levels with the same information, when possible)

_____ Attending to arrangement of material on page

_____ Providing highlighted texts/study guides

_____ Using supplementary materials

_____ Providing large-print materials

_____ Providing special equipment/assistive technology

_____ Highlighting important vocabulary, specific concepts, names, and dates prior to assigned reading

TEST TAKING

_____ Allowing open-book exams

_____ Giving exam orally

_____ Giving take-home tests

_____ Using more objective items (i.e., fewer essay responses)

_____ Allowing student to tape record test answers

_____ Giving frequent short quizzes, not long exams

_____ Allowing extra time for exams

_____ Reading test items to student

_____ Avoiding conditions of time or competition pressure

_____ Substituting a project for a test to demonstrate knowledge learned

_____ Providing someone to record student's answers

_____ Highlighting key words or phrases

_____ Allowing clarification on test questions as long as explanation does not give away the answers

_____ Eliminating computer-scored answer sheets

_____ Reducing number of choices on multiple-choice test

_____ Allowing tests to be taken in a separate, distraction-free environment

_____ Grading essay tests on content only; not penalized for spelling, capitalization, punctuation, or grammatical errors

_____ Allowing dictation of short answers to essay questions

_____ Providing key words for fill-in-the-blank tests

_____ Providing large-print tests

_____ *Additional accommodations:* _____

ORGANIZATION

_____ Providing peer assistance with organizational skills

_____ Assigning volunteer homework buddy

_____ Allowing student to have an extra set of books at home

_____ Sending daily or weekly progress reports home

(continued)

_____ Developing a reward system for in-school work and homework completion

_____ Providing student with a homework assignment notebook

_____ Providing proof reader

_____ Gathering progress reports from regular education teachers

_____ Providing a visual daily schedule

_____ Using study sheets to organize materials

_____ Using notebook with dividers

_____ Posting homework assignment in the same place

_____ Providing procedure for finished work

_____ Providing sample of finished product

_____ *Additional accommodations:* _____

BEHAVIORS

_____ Using timers to facilitate task completion

_____ Structuring transitional and unstructured times/places (e.g., recess, hallways, lunchroom, locker room, library, assembly, field trips, etc.)

_____ Praising specific behaviors

_____ Teaching self-monitoring strategies

_____ Giving extra privileges and rewards for acceptable behavior

_____ Keeping classroom rules simple and clear

_____ Making "prudent use" of negative consequences

_____ Allowing for short breaks between assignments

_____ Cueing student to stay on task (e.g., using a nonverbal signal)

_____ Marking student's correct answers, not mistakes

_____ Implementing a classroom behavior management system

_____ Allowing student time out of seat to run errands, etc.

_____ Ignoring inappropriate behaviors not drastically outside classroom limits

_____ Allowing legitimate movement

_____ Contracting with the student regarding expectations and rewards

_____ Increasing the immediacy of rewards

_____ Implementing time-out procedures

_____ Using timers to facilitate task completion

_____ Offering choices for responding to classroom demands

_____ *Additional accommodations:* _____

5

Integration/Reintegration into the School Setting

CHAPTER OBJECTIVES

It is essential for children with chronic illness to maintain their normal routines as much as possible, including when they are attending school. Adhering to routines helps children sustain both their academic progress and their social development. Because missing extended periods of school can have a detrimental impact on the academic and social development of children with chronic illness, getting them back to school is often a priority for the parents and the health care team. As previously discussed, integrating these children into the school environment can be very difficult, given their limitations and unique educational needs. This chapter addresses several issues associated with integrating or reintegrating children with chronic illness into the school environment. The list of issues discussed here is by no means exhaustive; I have included the most common ones faced by educators—those issues that often provide significant challenges to, or problems with, the process of appropriately including a child with chronic illness in day-to-day school activities. First I discuss the general issues and barriers involved in reintegration, then several specific issues and their recommendations for educators. Finally, I examine the development of an integration or reintegration plan using specific examples. The objectives of this chapter are:

- To review barriers associated with integration or reintegration into the school environment
- To discuss critical issues associated with integration
- To identify specific strategies for dealing with issues associated with integration
- To discuss the development of integration plans
- To illustrate the practical strategies for dealing with integration issues through the use of case examples

THE NEED FOR INTEGRATION

We now know that children with chronic illness must be integrated into the school environment, as dictated by law. Some children with a chronic illness do not miss school, and integrating them into the environment simply entails modifying their environment to fit their unique needs. However, school absence is common for many children with chronic illness, due to the effects of the illness as well as the treatments. Absences may be extended or short but frequent, unpredictable, and seemingly chronic. In cases of prolonged absence, special issues arise when the child returns to school. In either case, many obstacles and issues can prevent effective integration and produce stress and conflict for teachers, administrators, children, and their parents. The purpose of this chapter is to discuss issues that may be pertinent in both cases: reentry after initial diagnosis and treatment, as well as continued integration of children with longstanding chronic health conditions (e.g., diabetes or asthma).

OBSTACLES TO INTEGRATION

In their overview, Sexson and Madan-Swain (1993) do an excellent job of discussing many of the obstacles to school reentry faced by children with chronic illness and their. Here I summarize parts of their discussion, add examples of other obstacles from the literature and my own experiences, and provide specific examples.

ILLNESS AND TREATMENT EFFECTS

Many of the disease-specific symptoms of chronic illness make it impossible for children to attend school. These can include pain, deformity, nausea, fatigue, weakness, lethargy, susceptibility to infection, limited mobility, and cognitive impairment. Whereas some of these symptoms may make it physically impossible to attend school, others so significantly impact the child's ability to concentrate and participate that attending school is not an option. The disease may also alter the child's physical appearance in a manner that precludes the child from being seen by other children and adults.

In addition to the illness effects, negative effects of the treatment can also prevent children from attending school. In cases where treatment (e.g., chemotherapy) may compromise the immune system, children must be kept in a very controlled and isolated environment. In other cases the negative effects of treatments can include medication side effects, physically exhausting activities (e.g., physical therapy), physical deformity (e.g., amputation), and temporary or permanent physical and cognitive limitations. For example, medications that cause irritability and restlessness, cognitive impairment, sedation, or nausea can give rise to significant problems that prevent children from attending school. Table 5.1 contains a list of general barriers associated with illnesses and their treatment.

TABLE 5.1. Barriers to School Integration/Reintegration Resulting from Medical Conditions and Their Treatment

• Pain	• Compromised immune functioning
• Nausea	• Medication side effects
• Fatigue/weakness/exhaustion	• Cognitive impairment
• Physical deformity	• Limited mobility

Children's Issues

Many issues may serve as a barrier to children's participation in school. Children may experience social and/or emotional difficulties associated with their illness and treatment, such as those described above. They may be ashamed, scared, or fearful of what others might say or do, concerned about falling too far behind in their schoolwork, uneasy about feeling "different," anxious about separating from parents, and afraid of not knowing how to respond to the inquiries of the other children. In fact, as Sexson and Madan-Swain (1993) aptly point out, the immediate impact of delayed reentry may seem positive to the child. However, the delay ultimately reinforces the child's perceived hopelessness and unhealthy avoidant coping behavior.

In addition to social and emotional issues, children may have academic difficulties if they have missed many days of school. In most cases, children who have not had academic problems prior to the onset of their illness tend to do well in school once they have caught up on their studies. However, those who experience negative cognitive effects of the disease or its treatment may not be able to function at the same cognitive level as they did prior to the diagnosis and treatment. For example, children receiving cranial radiation for treatment of tumors may exhibit cognitive impairment that was not evident prior to their treatments. For such children, returning to school with these negative cognitive effects may be difficult, as both they and their parents fear academic failure. Children who experience learning problems prior to the diagnosis and treatment of their condition are at a greater risk for reentry problems. Sometimes there is a tendency for teachers to overlook a child's difficulties as due to the illness; therefore they do not believe that a referral to the school psychologist would be worthwhile. On the contrary, it is essential to identify and address these problems to prevent the child from becoming frustrated and experiencing accumulated academic failures (Sexson & Madan-Swain, 1993). Table 5.2 contains a list of children's issues that may form obstacles to school reentry.

TABLE 5.2. Children's Issues as Potential Barriers to School Integration/Reintegration

• Shame	• Fear of not knowing how to respond to peer inquiries
• Fear of being "different"	• Preillness learning problems
• Fear of what others might say or do	• Preillness social problems
• Concern about being too far behind in schoolwork	• Cognitive impairment
• Separation anxiety when separating from parents	

Adults' Issues

Parental attitudes can be critical to the successful integration of children with chronic illness into the school environment. Parents can be powerful advocates and sources of support for their children, but sometimes their own anxieties and attitudes can interfere with a successful integration process. Overprotectiveness, for example, can lead to a breakdown of appropriate expectations and boundaries for children, especially those who have a terminal illness. Additionally, the emotional and physical effort parents must exert to get a child back into a school routine can seem overwhelming when the child resists. In many cases, parents see school as a means to an academic outcome without recognizing its importance to the child's social development.

The attitudes of school personnel are obviously critical as well. Teachers and administrators are often uninformed and inexperienced at dealing with reentry issues and, in some cases, the difficult issues associated with continued integration. Likewise, teachers may feel overwhelmed, unsure of what to do, and uncomfortable dealing with the challenging issues that accompany these children. It is quite common for adults to experience difficulty dealing with significant child illnesses, particularly those that are terminal. (In Chapter 6 I discuss coping techniques for adults to use in dealing with their own concerns surrounding childhood illness and death.) Furthermore, teachers and administrators can feel overwhelmed by the needs of chronically ill children when they have limited resources to deal with their legal responsibilities. In such cases educators may become angry, resentful, and resistant when confronted with these comprehensive needs. Obviously, these attitudes are detrimental to the process of facilitating effective reintegration. Realistic expectations, effective communication, and mutual problem-solving efforts are necessary to overcome such barriers.

Finally, the health care team is key to effective reentry and integration. In many cases, it is what the health care team *does not* say that creates a barrier. The team should communicate clearly to the family that it is necessary for the child to return to school as soon as possible to further his or her social, developmental, and academic progress. Additionally, it is important for the health care team to establish effective means of communication with school staff. Often parents look to their child's physician for guidance on such matters as school integration. Unfortunately, physicians may not be well trained in education-specific issues, so it is critical that problem-solving efforts involve the parents and school officials as well. Table 5.3 lists adults' issues that may form barriers to reentry.

SPECIFIC ISSUES WITH INTEGRATION

This section addresses the many issues educators face when children with chronic illness are included in the general educational environment: for example, how to handle sensitive information about the child's condition, what to do about peer teasing, how to facilitate effective implementation of treatments in the school, and how to deal with activity restrictions.

TABLE 5.3. Adults' Issues as Potential Barriers to School Integration/Reintegration

- Parents' anxieties and overprotectiveness
- Parents' lowered expectations for their ill child
- Parents' lack of boundaries and discipline of child with illness
- Ongoing stress from child's illness reduces parents' ability to manage child's resistance to attending school
- School personnel overwhelmed by degree of children's needs and limited financial resources
- Teachers' anxieties and issues around loss and impending death
- Health care team's failure to emphasize the importance of return to school

Disclosure

One of the most difficult issues associated with integrating or reintegrating children with chronic illness into the classroom is the question of what to tell the other children. Since children are naturally curious, they are likely to ask questions of the teacher as well as the child with the illness. Curiosity is especially piqued when the child looks different as a result of the illness or its treatment, is not allowed to participate in all the activities, or has missed school on an extended basis. It is essential for both the child and the teacher to be prepared to answer questions to prevent adverse reactions of the other children, teasing of the ill child, or the problems that arise for teachers who discuss private issues without the consent of the child's parents.

Research has revealed that teachers have difficulties with taking on the role of educating children about another child's illness. For example, Eiser and Town (1987) surveyed 147 teachers and found that most limited their discussions to the causes and treatment of illnesses and what the children could do to help. Teachers also reported that they were likely to attempt any explanation only when they deemed it necessary, and few of the teachers saw it as their role to educate other children about illnesses. Less then 3% of the teachers felt able to discuss the possibility of the child's death. In many cases, teachers do not feel it is their responsibility, nor do they feel comfortable taking on the role of educating other children about the illness, despite it being a critical part of the ill child's integration into the classroom. Indeed, in a study of 58 families of children with chronic illness in the schools, the children expressed the need for teachers to help explain their condition to the other children (Mukherjee, Lightfoot, & Sloper, 2000).

Children with illness and their parents may or may not want other children and school officials to know about the disease. In Mukherjee and colleagues' (2000) study, the reasons children stated for wanting their peers to know about their condition included (1) knowing what to expect, (2) knowing what they (the peers) should do during a medical emergency, (3) knowing how to interact with the child (e.g., minimizing risk of infection), and (4) showing more empathy or understanding of the child's situation. Reasons for not wanting others to know included not wanting teachers to discuss personal or embarrassing matters in front of peers and preventing discrimination by other children or school officials and teasing.

Because of the varying desires of children and their families, it is very important that school officials discuss with the child and his or her parents exactly what they would like disclosed to other children and school personnel. Parents often find it difficult to balance their child's need to be treated "normally" with the need to disclose enough information to allow teachers to provide safe supervision (Bossert, Holaday, Harkins, & Turner-Henson, 1990). In addition to the ethical aspects of protecting the privacy of the child there are legal ones: School administrators may run into legal trouble by sharing information the family wishes to keep private. After clarifying what to disclose, school officials should also discuss when to disclose, how to disclose, and who should be involved in the disclosure process. Worksheet 5.1 (p. 74) contains a disclosure consent form to serve as guidance to teachers and serve as documentation as to the agreement between the child, his or her parents, and the school officials. In some cases the child may want the teacher to discuss the illness prior to the child's return. In other cases the child may actually want to be involved in the discussion of the illness, so that he or she can answer peers' questions with the help of the teacher.

Once an agreement has been reached about what to disclose, teachers and the child must be prepared to answer a wide range of questions. Table 5.4 contains a list of potential questions that teachers must be prepared to answer; you can see that there is a very wide range, and some of the questions may be difficult to answer. The issues get even more difficult when the child has a terminal illness, such as a brain tumor, and questions about the child's impending death arise. In any case, it is very important to talk with the children in developmentally appropriate terms. For example, it is important to avoid using abstract terms for younger children, because they will not understand. It is important to be direct and honest with children of all ages.

Worksheet 5.2 (p. 75) contains several questions that help parents and child to discuss these issues at home and formulate answers with which they are comfortable. Returning the completed worksheet to the school officials provides written documentation of family preferences. Figure 5.1 contains a completed worksheet for a third-grade boy with cancer who is returning to school following the first round of chemotherapy. You can see that the parents would like classmates to know about Johnny's condition, but they are not being explicit about the likelihood that he will die. These answers may change as Johnny's condition improves or worsens.

TABLE 5.4. Questions Typically Asked by Peers

- Is the disease contagious?
- Will _____ die from it?
- Will he/she lose any more limbs?
- Can _____ still play, visit me at home, drive, date, etc.?
- Should we talk about _____'s illness, or should we ignore it?
- What will other kids think if I'm still friends with _____?
- What's wrong with _____?
- Will _____ be different (look funny, bleed, faint, cough, vomit) when he/she comes back?

Note. From Sexson and Madan-Swain (1993). Copyright 1993 by Sage Publications, Inc. Reprinted by permission.

Your child has a medical condition that may prompt the questions of other children. Below are a list of potential questions that children may ask. Please complete the form to indicate how you would like school personnel to answer the questions if they arise about your child.

1. What is wrong with Johnny _____? He has a tumor in his head. _____

2. Why is he/she sick? Nobody knows for sure why Johnny got sick. _____

3. Can I catch the disease from Johnny _____? No, nobody can catch it from Johnny. _____

4. Is Johnny _____ going to die? We don't think so, but he is going to get very sick. _____

5. Can Johnny _____ still play with us? Yes, but he might get tired easily. _____

6. Will Johnny _____ keep missing school? He will miss school sometimes. _____

7. Why does Johnny _____ look funny? The treatment for his tumor makes his hair fall out. _____

8. Will Johnny _____ get better? In how long? We hope Johnny gets better, but we don't know for sure. _____

9. Why does he/she look so tired/sad? He doesn't feel good. _____

10. What can I do to help Johnny _____? Treat him like normal and be his friend. _____

11. What should I do if other kids pick on him/her? Tell them to stop and get the teacher. _____

12. Can I still be friends with Johnny _____? Yes, treat Johnny like you normally would. _____

13. When is Johnny _____ coming back to school? When he gets better, but we're not sure. _____

14. Should I talk about Johnny _____'s illness or not? You can ask Johnny what he wants. _____

15. Why can't Johnny _____ play in gym class with us? He is still sick, but will participate in other ways. _____

Other questions:

_____
_____
_____

| _____ | _____ | _____ | _____ |
| Parent Signature | Date | School Official | Date |

FIGURE 5.1. Completed Answering Questions about Your Child Worksheet.

Participation

An illness or its treatment can limit the type and amount of activities that a child can safely participate in during the school day. For example, a child with asthma or diabetes may be able to participate in physical education and sports activities with few limitations, given appropriate monitoring and medications. On the other hand, a child with severe juvenile rheumatoid arthritis may be so limited by pain and joint swelling that participation in physical education classes and sports is impossible. Likewise, children with heart abnormalities or bleeding disorders may not be allowed to engage in vigorous exercise in class or during recess. Limitations in activities may impact the child academically, and standing out from the other children can have significant social consequences. Being excluded from activities can make children feel ashamed, embarrassed, worthless, and inadequate. Inability to participate in activities may also increase the likelihood that the child will be teased or ridiculed by peers.

It is important for educators to understand the limitations resulting from medical conditions and creatively engage the ill child in appropriate and meaningful alternate ways. Mukherjee and colleagues (2000) reported that young people with chronic health conditions spoke enthusiastically about teachers who were sensitive to their needs and willing to adapt lessons so that they could participate in meaningful ways.

Determining if children can participate in physical education activities and sports is the first step in this phase. Table 5.5 contains general guidelines published by the American Academy of Pediatrics (2001) for determining whether children with specific medical conditions can participate in sports. This table can also help physical education instructors determine whether a particular student's participation in class activities is appropriate. In cases in which children cannot participate fully, it is essential that they be incorporated in some meaningful way, such as acting as scorekeeper or timekeeper (Sexson & Madan-Swain, 1993; Walsh & Ryan-Wenger, 1992), equipment manager, or coach. In one study, when modifications were necessary, youth reported preferring that teachers consult them about constructive alternative arrangements (Mukherjee et al., 2000).

In addition to physical education class, participation may become an issue in science classes (e.g., due to exposure to foreign substances), class trips (due to the need for medication storage and transfer, monitoring, need for mobility), and situations requiring extended school days (e.g., debate team, drama productions). Several factors may play a role in limiting the opportunities available to children with medical conditions to enjoy all the activities in school: fatigue associated with the illness or treatment, the need for specialized equipment, the need for access to emergency treatment, and limited mobility. It is important that educators recognize these limitations on participation, consult the affected children on ways to include them, and modify or adapt their course requirements so that these children can actively and meaningfully participate. Each child's physician and nurse are excellent sources of information, and their judgment regarding participation should weigh heavily in the decisions made regarding the child's level of participation.

TABLE 5.5. Medical Conditions and Sports Participation

Condition	May participate
Atlantoaxial instability (instability of the joint between cervical vertebrae 1 and 2)	Qualified yes

Explanation: Athlete needs evaluation to assess risk of spinal cord injury during sports participation.

Bleeding disorder	Qualified yes

Explanation: Athlete needs evaluation:

Cardiovascular disease

Carditis (inflammation of the heart)	No

Explanation: Carditis may result in sudden death with exertion.

Hypertension (high blood pressure)	Qualified yes

Explanation: Those with significant essential (unexplained) hypertension should avoid weight and power lifting, bodybuilding, and strength training. Those with secondary hypertension (hypertension caused by a previously identified disease) or severe essential hypertension need evaluation. The National High Blood Pressure Education Working group defined significant and severe hypertension.

Congenital heart disease (structural heart defects present at birth)	Qualified yes

Explanation: Those with mild forms may participate fully; those with moderate or severe forms or who have undergone surgery need evaluation. The 26th Bethesda Conference defined mild, moderate, and severe disease for common cardiac lesions.

Dysrhythmia (irregular heart rhythm)	Qualified yes

Explanation: Those with symptoms (chest pain, syncope, dizziness, shortness of breath, or other symptoms of possible dysrhythmia) or evidence of mitral regurgitation (leaking) on physical examination need evaluation. All others may participate fully.

Heart murmur	Qualified yes

Explanation: If the murmur is innocent (does not indicate heart disease), full participation is permitted. Otherwise, the athlete needs evaluation (*see* congenital heart disease and mitral valve prolapse).

Cerebral palsy	Qualified yes

Explanation: Athlete needs evaluation.

Diabetes mellitus	Yes

Explanation: All sports can be played with proper attention to diet, blood glucose concentration, hydration, and insulin therapy. Blood glucose concentration should be monitored every 30 minutes during continuous exercise and 15 minutes after completion of exercise.

Diarrhea	Qualified no

Explanation: Unless disease is mild, no participation is permitted, because diarrhea may increase the risk of dehydration and heat illness (*see* fever).

Eating disorders	Qualified yes

Anorexia nervosa
Bulimia nervosa

Explanation: Patients with these disorders need medical and psychiatric assessment before participation.

Eyes	Qualified yes

Functionally one-eyed athlete
Loss of an eye
Detached retina

(continued)

TABLE 5.5. (*continued*)

Condition	May participate
<u>Eyes</u> (*continued*)	
Previous eye surgery or serious eye injury	Qualified yes
Explanation: A functionally one-eyed athlete has a best-corrected visual acuity of less than 20/40 in the eye with worse acuity. These athletes would suffer significant disability if the better eye were seriously injured, as would those with loss of an eye. Some athletes who previously have undergone eye surgery or had a serious eye injury may have an increased risk of injury because of weakened eye tissue. Availability of eye guards approved by the American Society for Testing and Materials and other protective equipment may allow participation in most sports, but this must be judged on an individual basis.	
<u>Fever</u>	No
Explanation: Fever can increase cardiopulmonary effort, reduce maximum exercise capacity, make heat illness more likely, and increase orthostatic hypertension during exercise. Fever may rarely accompany myocarditis or other infections that may make exercise dangerous.	
<u>Heat illness, history of</u>	Qualified yes
Explanation: Because of the increased likelihood of recurrence, the athlete needs individual assessment to determine the presence of predisposing conditions and to arrange a prevention strategy.	
<u>Hepatitis</u>	Yes
Explanation: Because of the apparent minimal risk to others, all sports may be played that the athlete's state of health allows. In all athletes, skin lesions should be covered properly, and athletic personnel should use universal precautions when handling blood or body fluids with visible blood.	
<u>Human immunodeficiency virus infection</u>	Yes
Explanation: Because of the apparent minimal risk to others, all sports may be played that the athlete's state of health allows. In all athletes, skin lesions should be covered properly, and athletic personnel should use universal precautions when handling blood or body fluids with visible blood.	
<u>Kidney, absence of one</u>	Qualified yes
Explanation: Athlete needs individual assessment for contact, collision, and limited-contact sports.	
<u>Liver, enlarged</u>	Qualified yes
Explanation: If the liver is acutely enlarged, participation should be avoided because of risk of rupture. If the liver is chronically enlarged, individual assessment is needed before collision, contact, or limited-contact sports are played.	
<u>Malignant neoplasm</u>	Qualified yes
Explanation: Athlete needs individual assessment.	
<u>Musculoskeletal disorders</u>	Qualified yes
Explanation: Athlete needs individual assessment.	
<u>Neurological disorders</u>	
History of serious head or spine trauma, severe or repeated concussions, or crainotomy.	Qualified yes
Explanation: Athlete needs individual assessment for collision, contact, or limited-contact sports and also for noncontact sports if deficits in judgment or cognition are present. Research supports a conservative approach to management of concussion.	
Seizure disorder, well-controlled	Yes
Explanation: Risk of seizure during participation is minimal.	*(continued)*

TABLE 5.5. *(continued)*

Condition	May participate
<u>Neurological disorders</u> *(continued)*	
Seizure disorder, poorly controlled	Qualified yes
Explanation: Athlete needs individual assessment for collision, contact, or limited-contact sports. The following noncontact sports should be avoided: archery, riflery, swimming, weight or power lifting, strength training, or sports involving heights. In these sports, occurrence of a seizure may pose a risk to self or others.	
Obesity	Qualified yes
Explanation: Because of the risk of heat illness, obese persons need careful acclimatization and hydration.	
<u>Organ transplant recipient</u>	Qualified yes
Explanation: Athlete needs individual assessment.	
<u>Ovary, absence of one</u>	Yes
Explanation: Risk of severe injury to the remaining ovary is minimal.	
<u>Respiratory conditions</u>	
Pulmonary compromise, including cystic fibrosis	Qualified yes
Explanation: Athlete needs individual assessment, but generally, all sports may be played if oxygenation remains satisfactory during a graded exercise test. Patients with cystic fibrosis need acclimatization and good hydration to reduce the risk of heat illness.	
Asthma	Yes
Explanation: With proper medication and education, only athletes with the most severe asthma will need to modify their participation.	
Acute upper respiratory infection	Qualified yes
Explanation: Upper respiratory obstruction may affect pulmonary function. Athlete needs individual assessment for all but mild disease *(see* fever).	
<u>Sickle cell disease</u>	Qualified yes
Explanation: Athlete needs individual assessment. In general, if status of the illness permits, all but high exertion, collision, and contact sports may be played. Overheating, dehydration, and chilling must be avoided.	
<u>Sickle cell trait</u>	Yes
Explanation: It is unlikely that persons with sickle cell trait have an increased risk of sudden death or other medical problems during athletic participation, except under the most extreme conditions of heat, humidity, and possibly increased altitude. These persons, like all athletes, should be carefully conditioned, acclimatized, and hydrated to reduce any possible risk.	
<u>Skin disorders</u> (boils, herpes simplex, impetigo, scabies, molluscum contagiosum)	Qualified yes
Explanation: While the patient is contagious, participation in gymnastics with mats, martial arts, wrestling, or other collision, contact, or limited-contact sports is not allowed.	
<u>Spleen, enlarged</u>	Qualified yes
Explanation: A patient with an acutely large spleen should avoid all sports because of risk of rupture. A patient with a chronically enlarged spleen needs individual assessment before playing collision, contact, or limited-contact sports.	
<u>Testicle, undescended or absence of one</u>	Yes
Explanation: Certain sports may require a protective cup.	

Teasing/Bullying

Children with chronic illness often look or act differently from their peers, due to the effects of the illness or its treatment. In many cases, being different from the "norm" means that these children are victims of teasing, ridicule, and bullying. Mukherjee and colleagues (2000) reported that over a third of the children with chronic illness in their study reported being teased or bullied and expressed a desire for their teachers to intervene. Teasing and bullying may take the forms of verbal harassment (name calling, threats), practical jokes, and public ridicule regarding personal issues associated with the illness or its treatment (e.g., baldness, the need for specialized equipment, inability to participate). In addition to outright bullying, these children are often ignored altogether by their peers, resulting in social isolation. In any case, it is the responsibility of educators to deal directly and swiftly with these issues.

A thorough description of bullying behaviors and methods for preventing and dealing with them in schools is clearly beyond the scope of this chapter. Nonetheless, the importance of dealing with bullying cannot be overstated. Table 5.6 lists additional resources for dealing with bullying in the schools in general. I encourage all teachers to gather informational resources to address this important topic. Teachers and parents should take a proactive approach to dealing with the potential for teasing or bullying. If necessary, 504 plans or IEPs should contain a specific plan for dealing with social isolation, teasing, or bullying directly and swiftly, before secondary problems, such as fear of returning to school or anxiety/depression, develop. Handout 5.1 (p. 76) is a document designed to help parents and educators deal with bullying. It contains specific suggestions to help children with behavioral responses when they are the victim of bullying. Teasing is discussed further in Chapter 6, which also contains several additional worksheets.

TABLE 5.6. Additional Resources for Dealing with Bullying and Teasing in Schools

Banks, R. (1998). *What should parents and teachers know about bullying?* Washington, DC: U.S. Educational Resources Information Center. http:www.edrs.com/members/ericfac.cfm?an=ED424037

Ericson, N. (2001). *Addressing the problem of juvenile bullying.* Washington, DC: U.S. Department of Justice, Office of Juvenile Justice and Delinquency Prevention.

Juvonen, J., & Graham, S. (Eds.). (2001). *Peer harassment in school: The plight of the vulnerable and victimized.* New York: Guilford Press.

Olweus, D. (1999). *Bullying prevention program.* Boulder: Center for the Study and Prevention of Violence, Institute of Behavioral Science, University of Colorado.

Sampson, R. (2002). Bullying in schools. In *Problem-oriented guides for police series* (No. 12). Washington, DC: U.S. Department of Justice, Office of Community Oriented Policing Services. *http:// purl.access.gpo.gov/GPO/LPS19843*

Sullivan, K. (2000). *The anti-bullying handbook.* New York: Oxford University Press.

CONCLUDING COMMENTS

This chapter discusses many of the issues associated with reentry and reintegration. Handout 5.2 (p. 77) is a guide for parents to aid in the reentry process. Educators may be well served by photocopying the handout and providing a copy to parents. More detailed descriptions of how to deal with reentry issues are contained in subsequent chapters.

WORKSHEET 5.1. Consent Form for Disclosure

Your child has a medical condition that may affect him/her in school. Naturally, children may ask questions about your child's condition. You may wish to share this information with your child's peers and school personnel, or you may wish to keep this information private. There are advantages and disadvantages to each choice. Please indicate below whether you would like information disclosed about your child's condition. If you would like information to be disclosed, please describe your wishes below.

_____ **Yes**, you have permission to discuss my child's condition with other school personnel and my child's peers.

_____ **Yes**, you have permission to discuss my child's condition with other school personnel but **not** my child's peers.

_____ **No**, we would like to keep my child's condition private. Please **do not** disclose information about my child's medical condition with anyone in the school.

If yes, please describe below what you would like disclosed.

_____

_____

_____

_____

Please describe below how you would like this information shared with others.

_____

_____

_____

_____

_____   _____   _____   _____
Parent Signature   Date   School Official   Date

WORKSHEET 5.2. Answering Questions about Your Child

Your child has a medical condition that may prompt the questions of other children. Below are a list of potential questions that children may ask. Please complete the form to indicate how you would like school personnel to answer the questions if they arise about your child.

1. What is wrong with _____? _____

2. Why is he/she sick? _____

3. Can I catch the disease from _____? _____

4. Is _____ going to die? _____

5. Can _____ still play with us? _____

6. Will _____ keep missing school? _____

7. Why does _____ look funny? _____

8. Will _____ get better? In how long? _____

9. Why does he/she look so tired/sad? _____

10. What can I do to help _____? _____

11. What should I do if other kids pick on him/her? _____

12. Can I still be friends with _____? _____

13. When is _____ coming back to school? _____

14. Should I talk about _____'s illness or not? _____

15. Why can't _____ play in gym class with us? _____

Other questions:

_____

_____

_____

Parent Signature	Date	School Official	Date

HANDOUT 5.1. Helping Children Handle Teasing

At some point or another, almost all children have to endure teasing from friends, classmates, siblings, etc. For many children, teasing by others is a temporary thing, and they are able to handle it with a minimum amount of difficulty. For other children, however, teasing is more frequent. Some children are more vulnerable to teasing than others, and are singled out for frequent teasing by peers. This may be because the child looks different from his or her peers, acts differently, or responds to the teasing in a way that encourages more teasing. When teasing is frequent, the victim needs your help. Teasing can be very painful for children, and it can affect their self-esteem and how they relate to other people. The best thing that you can do to help children who are being teased is to teach constructive ways to respond to teasing. Here are some things you can do to help children handle teasing.

Gather information. First, try to find out some specifics about the situation from the child: for example, what the teasing is about, who is doing the teasing, where the teasing is occurring, how the child is reacting to different episodes, and what occurs afterward. Try to keep track of this type of information for a few days to find out what precipitates the teasing and if there seems to be some pattern to it.

Talk about appropriate responses. There are two basic ways in which children can respond to teasing without teasing back:
- *Ignore it.* Many teasers quickly give up when they find they have no audience. Teach the child to ignore the teasing by turning and walking away without saying a word. Make sure the child knows that at first the teaser may try even harder to get a response out of him or her, and that it is important to hold his or her ground and not respond. It should not take long before the teaser gives up.
- *Develop a quick tongue.* Sometimes a quick response will throw a teaser off track. It is important, however, that this quick response *not* be in the form of teasing back or name calling. If the taunts are often the same from day to day, parents can teach their children specific responses. For example, to the tease "Your mother wears combat boots," the child could reply something like "That's silly, my mother doesn't even own a pair of boots." Or, if the taunts differ, the child could say something like "I know you're trying to upset me, and it's not going to work, no matter what you do."

Practice. It is important to practice with the children whatever responses you come up with together. Role play the situation. Try saying things to the child the way the teaser does, and have the child practice his or her responses. This exercise not only helps children get used to the teasing, but as a result of practice, the teasing is experienced as less upsetting. This also helps children develop appropriate ways of responding to the teasing. The more children practice appropriate responses, the more likely they will be to use them when they are teased.

Provide lots of support and encouragement. Once the child comes up with a method that works, support him or her in these efforts. Make sure to tell the child just how proud you are when he or she attempts to resolve teasing situations appropriately.

Remember that at some point or another, all children are teased. In cases where children are very sensitive to it, or the teasing goes on for a period of time, it is up to the adults to intervene in some way to help children learn to cope.

HANDOUT 5.2. A Parent's Guide to School Reentry

Children and adolescents with a chronic (e.g., diabetes) or life-threatening (e.g., cancer) illness who return to school following their diagnosis and initial treatment are faced with many challenges. Changes in body image, daily medication needs, fatigue related to the illness or treatment, and social isolation due to hospitalization are a few examples of complications to a smooth transition back to school. However, there are accommodations that can be initiated to make school reentry less taxing. Some examples include a shortened school day, assistance with note taking, or special equipment to assist learning.

The return to school can be made smoother with early planning and good communication between the school, the student and family, and the medical team. Inform the principal as soon as you know when your child will return to school. Next, contact the school nurse, homeroom and other teachers, and counselor so they can prepare for the child's return. It is critical that parents keep the school informed when there are changes in their child's condition that might affect educational progress, and that they actively communicate any concerns they or their child have about school reentry. Understanding the roles of the following health and educational professionals will help in this process:

- **School nurse:** Whether or not the school nurse works at the school every day, he or she is trained to understand complex medical conditions and translate the educational implications to the school team.
- **Principal:** Keep the principal informed of all actions taken on behalf of your child. He or she knows the regulations of the state and policies of the school district, as well as the necessary authority structure to obtain accommodations.
- **School psychologist:** The school psychologist accesses special education services for your child and participates in the development of individualized education plans and Section 504 plans (see below).
- **School counselor:** The school counselor is knowledgeable about the many social, emotional, and academic resources in the school district and often has experience with students who need accommodations. Counselors monitor credits needed for graduation and can also determine alternative educational options if the regular school setting is not appropriate.
- **Home/hospital tutor:** The school district can arrange for home or hospital tutoring. Parents need to obtain a doctor's letter stating that their child is unable to attend school; they may also need to write a formal parental request for a home tutor. Although home tutor policies are different in each district, it is common for a tutor to be assigned to a child for 2 hours per day for every day the student is expected to miss school. Apply early; many school districts have a minimum absence period (e.g., 2 weeks), and it can take time to find a home tutor. If shorter but frequent absences are likely due to the health condition, provide a physician-signed letter explaining your child's medical circumstances and obtain a commitment for tutoring on an intermittent basis. This arrangement may require a 504 plan (see below).
- **Primary nurse:** This hospital or clinic-based liaison should convey essential medical information to the school personnel in a timely fashion (with written parental permission), since there are often rapid changes in medications, medication schedules, or medical treatments during therapy that can affect school participation.

(continued)

THE LAW

There are educational laws that ensure that children get the help they need when special services and accommodations are necessary. Parents or guardians must give permission before any accommodations can be made at school, including changes in the school day.

- The **Individuals with Disabilities Education Act (IDEA)** provides for special education services for eligible students. The most common type of educational disability for children with a chronic illness is categorized as "other health impaired," which means that the child's health status is having a negative impact on learning.
- An **individualized education plan (IEP)** is written when special education services are needed. An IEP is reviewed annually, although it is in force for 3 years, and the assessment is performed every 3 years. If your child is 14 years or older, the IEP should include a "transition plan" that includes steps to making the transition to the workplace or higher education after graduation. An example of a transition plan is one that provides for vocational training during high school in the student's chosen career.
- **Section 504** provides for nondiscrimination and equal access to educational opportunities for students with disabilities. A 504 plan can be written to include accommodations such as a shortened school day, testing modifications, or an extra set of books at home. The 504 plan is in force for 1 year and is renewed as necessary.

School districts have many resources and services that can help children return to school with a chronic illness or after a life-threatening illness; in general, school personnel are eager to help. Strive for open and honest communication with the involved health and educational professionals to ensure that your child's experience is successful. This approach also increases the likelihood that school personnel will remain as flexible as possible so that the school continues to be a positive experience for the returning student. In addition, encourage your child to talk with medical and school personnel when needed. Children can be their own best advocates. They, alone, know how tired they are and the limits of their capacity for schoolwork, socialization, and learning. Be sure they know how to contact the school psychologist and guidance counselor if any problems arise while at school, such as issues with peers or teachers. It is important for returning students to feel that there is support available on site.

INTERNET RESOURCES

<u>Starbright Foundation</u>

This site is dedicated to developing projects that help chronically ill children and teens overcome the medical and emotional challenges they face. It offers several videos for preteens and teens, including how to communicate with the doctor and the hospital staff, as well as one entitled *Back to School: Teens Prepare for School Re-Entry.* The videos are free to families of children with a chronic or life-threatening illness. The back-to-school video also contains a resource manual that discusses the law and suggests possible accommodations. The website also includes links to other sites that provide information on various medical procedures and conditions.

While I do not endorse any of the following websites, they are listed here because they provide educational resources for children with chronic or life-threatening illnesses. The titles in italics are pamphlets that can be downloaded or ordered from the organization.

(continued)

American Cancer Society (www.cancer.org)
Teachers of Children with Cancer

American Diabetes Association (www.diabetes.org)
Your School and Your Rights
The ABC's of Managing Diabetes at School

American Heart Association (www.americanheart.org)
School Programs
Your Child's Special Needs

Aplastic Anemia and MDS (Myelodysplastic Syndromes) International Foundation, Inc.
(www.aplastic.org)

Candlelighters Childhood Cancer Foundation (www.candlelighters.org)
Educating the Child with Cancer

Children's Liver Association for Support Services (www.classkids.org)

Crohn's and Colitis Foundation of America (www.ccfa.org)
A Teachers Guide to Crohn's Disease & Ulcerative Colitis

Cystic Fibrosis Foundation (www.cff.org)
Teachers Guide to CF

Epilepsy Foundation (www.epilepsyfoundation.org)
Making Our Schools Seizure Smart: Introduction
Making Our Schools Seizure Smart: Seizures and School
Making Our Schools Seizure Smart: Seizure Prevention
Making Our Schools Seizure Smart: School Performance
Making Our Schools Seizure Smart: Seizure Recognition
Making Our Schools Seizure Smart: Managing Seizures at School

Leukemia Lymphoma Society (www.leukemia-lymphoma.org)
Why Charlie Brown, Why? [video]
Cancervive
Making the Grade [video]
Back to School curriculum

National Brain Tumor Foundation (www.braintumor.org)
Your Child's Brain Tumor [extensive section on education]

National Cancer Institute (http://cis.nci.nih.gov)
Cancer Facts
Students with Cancer
Cancer Net (www.cancer.gov/cancerinformation)

6

Coping with Chronic Health Conditions

with RAELYNN MALONEY *and* JAMI GROSS

CHAPTER OBJECTIVES

When compared to their healthy peers, children with chronic health conditions are at increased risk of experiencing adjustment problems, including behavior problems, emotional distress such as sadness and anger, difficulty in social relationships, social anxiety, negative self-image, and poor school performance (Cohen, 1999). However, despite these increased risks, many of these children are able to avoid such problems and adjust quite well to the challenges that accompany their diagnosis. You may find that identifying a student who is having difficulty with adjustment can be a challenging role. It may, however, be the most significant role you play in the life of a student with a chronic health condition. Every day there are opportunities for you to offer various types of support to these students as they manage the practical and emotional challenges associated with their health conditions. You play a unique role as a social resource for these children, providing help directly as well as indirectly. For example, you may be in a position to help a student to remember his or her medication routine. You may assist fellow school personnel in creating an intervention plan to obtain accommodations that will improve the child's school experience. A child may need your guidance to cope with a problematic social situation or to appreciate positive comments received from someone he or she respects (e.g., a teacher, coach, or counselor) about something he or she is doing well. It is also likely that children with chronic illness will seek some form of support from you that they do not, cannot, or

Raelynn Maloney, MA, Psychological and Quantitative Foundations, University of Iowa, Iowa City, Iowa
Jami Gross, BA, Psychological and Quantitative Foundations, University of Iowa, Iowa City, Iowa

are not willing to obtain from others. Handout 6.1 (p. xx) contains additional examples of the kinds of tasks you can perform to help these students.

With your encouragement and guidance, children with health problems can learn to navigate the coping process and manage environmental and health-related stressors in the school setting with greater ease. *A stressor is any circumstance or object that is perceived as a potential threat to one's physical, psychological, or social well-being.* In this chapter we provide the information and tools you will need to assist children who are having difficulty coping. The chapter is divided into two sections. The first section covers the coping process, factors that influence coping, how to identify students who need help, and how to teach children effective ways of coping with a variety of stressors. The second section is designed to facilitate your personal coping and enhance your own ability to integrate self-care into your daily routine. The specific objectives of this chapter are:

- To define and discuss concepts related to children's coping
- To help you identify children who may need help coping
- To provide you with tools to help children with health conditions cope better with their illnesses
- To help you assess your own coping
- To teach you skills to cope with personal and work-related stressors

HELPING STUDENTS COPE

Regardless of their health status, all children must confront the developmental tasks and challenges of childhood and adolescence as they mature. Mastering the socioemotional tasks associated with any particular developmental period, such as establishing independence and intimate relationships during adolescence, is as important for a child who is living with a chronic health condition as it is for his or her peers. By the same token, no child can escape the day-to-day challenges that are a natural part of growing up. Children and adolescents are not immune to experiencing daily life hassles. *Daily hassles are those slight misfortunes that create ripples or interference in the flow of your day or week.* For students, daily hassles might include disagreements with friends, losing lunch money, forgetting to do an assignment, missing the bus, getting hurt on the playground, or dealing with the pain and impairment of a health condition. Despite how much their lives appear to resemble their peers, it is important to recognize that the daily experiences of students with health conditions may differ in many important ways from those who are without similar health-related challenges. Although this awareness is especially difficult to retain when the child's health condition is invisible (e.g., asthma, kidney disease), it is essential if you are to understand the unique concerns and needs of these children. Consider, for a moment, the small but significant lifestyle changes that occur when certain health conditions arise, such as modifications in daily schedules and self-care routines. A child who is diabetic, for instance, must incorporate medical tasks (e.g., blood glucose monitoring, insulin injections) into his or her daily routine, regardless of how this interferes with learning, disrupts play, or creates discomfort while interacting with peers. The child with asthma is strongly encouraged to avoid certain situations or environments wherein he or she may be exposed to harmful allergens; for this child, even a simple field trip becomes an event that requires careful consideration and planning. The child who is required to take medications several times each day may be a child whose inflexibly scheduled meals may result in many missed opportunities to eat lunch with his or her best friend. Table 6.1 lists common daily stressors for all children and additional stressors unique to children who have health-related conditions.

What Stressors Do Children with Health Conditions Face?

In addition to lifestyle modifications, many of the common problems that are experienced by many children, at least some of the time, tend to occur more often and more intensely for children who have health-related stressors. For instance, children living with chronic health conditions generally miss more days of school than their healthy peers, because of illness-related symptoms, medical treatments, treatment side effects, or hospitalizations. Learning difficulties may develop or previously existing learning problems may become aggravated by the disease process or medical interventions. Some treatments, such as radiation and certain medications, have a direct impact on children's central nervous system, rendering these children vulnerable to learning difficulties. Doctors or concerned parents may feel the need to restrict children with specific health conditions from participation in age-appropriate school and social activities. Not only are these children faced with threats to their physical health brought on by the disease itself, but at the same time they must cope with the emotional and social implications as well. Children show a wide variety of emotions about their disease progression and potential death, including relief, reassurance, uncertainty, concern, or fear. Children's social lives can be dramatically altered by illness as well. They may spend more time away from school and thus less time engaged in the daily social activities at school. Depending on the child's diagnosis and other familial factors, parents may be overprotective and strict about the child's involvement in certain social activities. What's more, many chronically ill children are confronted with the added stress of perceiving their parents' fears, shame, embarrassment, or concerns about how the disease is impacting their growth, mood, peer and family relationships, school performance, or quality of life. A list of these and other health-related stressors is provided in Table 6.2.

TABLE 6.1. Common and Health-Specific Daily Stressors for Students

Common stressors	Disease/health-related stressors
Homework	Undergoing treatments
Fighting with siblings	Missing school due to illness
Getting a bad grade	Pain
Arguing with parents	Missing social activities
Losing a friend	Being in the hospital
Losing lunch money	Being teased about illness
Being late for school	Sitting out during recess or physical education

TABLE 6.2 Examples of Health-Related Stressors

Medical

    Integrating medical tasks into daily routine
    Managing a complex medication regimen
    Lifestyle modifications (e.g., eating restrictions,
        exercise restrictions, sleep difficulties)

Physical

    Growth suppression
    Changes in physical appearance
    Intermittent or chronic pain

Academic

    Absence from school and social activities
    Decline in academic performance
    Development or exacerbation of learning difficulties

Psychological

    Somatic responses
    Losses associated with illness (e.g.,
        eyesight, limbs, hair)
    Uncertain future
    End-of-life concerns

Social

    Environmental precautions
    Restrictions in freedom and activities
    Changes in the parent–child relationship
    Changes in peer relationships

A Review of Coping Concepts

Coping has been defined many ways in the scientific literature. One of the most familiar definitions was initially proposed by Lazarus and Folkman (1984) and later elaborated by Spirito, Stark, and Tyc (1995). These experts define coping as *the active and intentional use of cognitive and behavioral strategies to help mediate a stressful situation.* Although the terms are often used interchangeably, it is important to keep in mind that "coping with illness" is not synonymous with "adaptation to illness." *Adaptation* is a broad term often used to refer more generally to overall outcome or adjustment to a situation; *coping* is one of many aspects of adaptation. Coping is what children actively engage to attain adaptation. When presented with a situation that is perceived as stressful, using effective coping skills makes it easier for the person to adapt well to the situation.

Coping Style

Adults tend to employ firmly established ways of approaching stressful situations. Strategies are less fixed, however, for children, and often differ depending on the type of stressor (e.g., whether it is disease-related versus non-disease-related) or the context of the situation (e.g., during school versus at home). Children may also use different coping strategies when the stressor is perceived to be within their control versus uncontrollable. The range of coping strategies that a child uses will ultimately develop, with experience, into a pattern of coping that becomes his or her coping style. A coping style is *a person's inclination to respond to a range of stressful situations in a particular way* (Boekaerts & Roder, 1999). The good news is that children can be taught new and positive ways of coping to more effectively manage the stresses of illness. This means that even if a child has established a way of coping that is not beneficial, professionals such as yourself can help him or her develop a more effective coping style by teaching new and more effective coping strategies.

Approach versus Avoidant Coping

Coping styles are often categorized as either approach or avoidant coping, with the primary difference being the focus of the strategies (Boekaerts & Roder, 1999). Researchers have found differences in the coping styles used by different children. Children who use approach coping aim their coping attempts *directly at* the stressor. For example, a child may read about his or her disease to better understand it and therefore reduce the mystery surrounding it or the fears associated with it. Avoidant coping, on the other hand, involves strategies directed *away from* the stressor. A child who uses avoidant coping may choose to read a magazine instead of listening to the physician talk about the progression of his or her disease. Although some avoidant strategies may be helpful during periods of acute stress, overall, children who have an approach coping style deal better with the stress of a chronic illness, researchers report (Meijer, Sinnema, Bijstra, Mellenbergh, & Wolters, 2002). Many of the adjustment difficulties discussed previously are often linked with the overuse of avoidant and passive coping strategies, such as social withdrawal, wishful thinking, and inactively waiting for things to get better. Researchers have observed that healthy adjustment and increased self-confidence are more often associated with the use of active approaches (Boekaerts & Roder, 1999), such as seeking emotional or informational support, talking about problems with others, asking for help, exploring options, developing a plan of action, making decisions, or confronting the issue directly. For example, a student who is being teased during recess may ask the playground monitor how to make the teasers stop. Or, following diagnosis, a child and his or her parents may search the Internet or bookstore shelves to find a quality resource to learn more about the disease and its treatment. A student may ask his or her teacher or parent if there is a support group for kids "like him"/"like her" who are living with cystic fibrosis (or asthma, juvenile rheumatoid arthritis, etc.).

Problem-Focused versus Emotion-Focused Coping

Coping styles can also be categorized as problem-focused or emotion-focused, based on their function. In problem-focused coping, a child attempts to *change the stressor* itself. Emotion-focused coping, on the other hand, is used as an attempt to *deal with the emotions* related to the stressor. For example, if Billy's peers have given him a nickname because of his hair loss, he may anticipate their teasing and develop a specific response of asking them to stop. This is an example of problem-focused coping. He may also go to his teacher during recess to talk about how the nickname hurts his feelings—an example of emotion-focused coping.

Coping Strategies

The ways in which children cope with daily life and health-related stressors are as diverse as the illnesses they confront. Every chronic illness or health condition is approached and handled in a different way by different children. As discussed earlier, one of the factors that influences the way a child approaches a particular life stressor, or set of stressors, is his or her *coping style*. A second influential factor is the body of *coping strategies* that the child has adopted to manage feelings of distress and reestablish a sense of safety and control. A coping strategy is *a response to a distressing situation that alters the situation or the person's perception of the situation in such a way that it is no longer distressing* (Lazarus & Folkman, 1984). Lists of cognitive and behavioral coping strategies that you may observe children using can be found in Tables 6.3 and 6.4, respectively. Although these lists are thorough, they are by no means exhaustive. With this in mind, we invite you to add items to this list based on your own observations.

Cognitive Appraisal

You may ask, "What internal process determines how a particular stressor will be approached?" The emotions that are stirred when a child is presented with or confronts a stressor affect the way he or she thinks about the stressor. For children with chronic illness, feelings about the illness influence their attitudes, perceptions, and beliefs about the illness. Cognitive appraisal is the *process through which a person, guided by his or her emotional responses to a situation, generates thoughts about, and makes meaning of, the situation* (Lazarus & Folkman, 1984). Researchers have shown that the way in which children make sense of the stress in their lives helps them to organize the experience in their own mind, and in turn influences the way they choose to deal with the stress. According to Lazarus and Folkman (1984), children make two types of appraisals: (1) an appraisal about the threat or risk of the stressor (i.e., "How will this affect me?") and (2) an appraisal of their capacity to handle the stressor (i.e., "What can I do about this?"). For example, Cindy worried that she would not be able to play her favorite sport because she was diagnosed with severe asthma during summer break—an appraisal of threat or risk. She also made an appraisal of her personal capacity to manage the stressor when she realized that she could

TABLE 6.3. Cognitive Coping Strategies

Cognitive methods	Examples
Denial—Attempts to deny the existence of a stressor	Daydreaming; ignoring your pain; minimizing the significance of the situation (e.g., "It's no big deal")
Distraction—Refocuses or diverts your attention away from a stressor	Avoids thinking about the pain; wishful thinking about the pain disappearing; distracting yourself with humor or an activity such as reading, listening to music
Cognitive restructuring—Changes your perception or the way you think about the stressor	Positively reframing the pain as temporary and tolerable; positive self-talk
Problem solving—Examines the problem and develops ways of responding to it that alter the situation; think about ways to modify, prevent, or eliminate a stressor	Planning, accepting responsibility, problem solving
Think ahead—Anticipates problems and plans ahead	Expect to experience the pain and prepare what you will say to yourself or aloud in response to the pain ahead of time

TABLE 6.4. Behavioral Coping Strategies

Behavioral methods	Examples
Engages in an activity that puts distance between you and the stressor or thoughts about the stressor	Listening to music, watching television
Learns more about the stressor	Talking to others about the stressor including family, school personnel, medical team, religious leaders, or others; using Internet resources; gaining information from television, books, or other sources
Engages in behaviors that may isolate you from others	Playing alone; having poor hygiene; withdrawing from social activities or groups
Accepts support from others who care about you and that you respect	Talking to and receiving guidance from family, friends, teachers, coaches, or others
Participates in activities that give you a sense of self-control or help you to manage your emotions	Using relaxation exercises; guided imagery; yoga; journaling
Seeks spiritual support	Using prayer; meditation
Attempts to alter the situation by aggressive means	Engaging in verbal or physical acting out; taking your anger or frustration out on someone else with words or physical force; engaging in destructive behaviors such as destroying property

continue to participate as long as she takes the necessary precautions, such as keeping her inhaler nearby in case she has an asthma attack.

The emotional meaning that children give to their health condition, and to any other stressor, changes as a function of gender and age (Band & Weisz, 1990; Spirito et al., 1995). For girls, the strain that disease and illness puts on close relationships is often more difficult for them to manage than it is for boys, especially as they approach adolescence. For example, a teenage girl is more likely than a teenage boy to talk about feeling guilty for being sick because it makes her less available to a friend who really needs support after a relationship breakup. Researchers have also found that because of differences in cognitive, emotional, and social development, a child's age can be very influential in shaping his or her coping responses (Meijer et al., 2002). Handout 6.2 (p. 129) highlights these developmental differences in coping. Children's ability to process stress and articulate their experience is a function of age, cognitive capacity, emotional development, previous successes, temperament, and problem-solving ability, among other factors. For example, a third grader may talk about feeling sad about having to miss school for a period of time to go back into the hospital, whereas an adolescent is more likely to describe frustration with the social interference of hospitalization.

Children's coping style and available coping skills are essentially products of past experiences in which they interact with, and witness the coping styles and strategies of, parents, siblings, peers, teachers, coaches, and other role models. For example, a child may be encouraged by his or her parents to approach a difficult situation the way they would (e.g., "Just ignore their comments," "Walk away"). A child may also observe and appraise a peer's success or failure when using a particular strategy (e.g., ignoring) when being teased and choose to approach the situation differently (e.g., ask a teacher for help) if the outcome was negative.

Children also develop adaptive or maladaptive views of their illness primarily based on familial influences, although it is quite possible that other well-respected individuals can encourage the adoption of adaptive "illness representations" (Lau, Quadrel, & Hartman, 1990). If Lisa's illness is represented in her mind as an enemy or a weakness, she may experience a diminished sense of hope and feel discouraged or cynical about her prospects. On the other hand, if she perceives her illness as a surmountable challenge or as simply a part of who she is, her approach to illness-related stressors would likely be more adaptive. She may have fewer negative appraisals of her ability to handle stressors and be more willing to ask for guidance from others. Illness representations have been shown to greatly influence a child's ability to cope with and adapt to illness (Lau, Quadrel, & Hartman, 1990). Table 6.5 provides definitions of the terms associated with theories and methods of coping.

The Coping Process

Figure 6.1 presents the coping concepts discussed so far (i.e., stressors, cognitive appraisal processes, coping strategy, and adaptation). This visual diagram represents the general flow of children's coping experiences. We use this model as a scaffold upon which we design a more complete image, and thus a more thorough understanding, of the coping experience of students who have chronic health conditions.

Take note of the pattern of flow in the model. The process begins when a child experiences something stressful (which may or may not be related to his or her illness). The child mentally and emotionally processes the stressor by (1) experiencing the stressor, (2) appraising the threat of the situation and his or her ability to manage this threat, (3) emotionally responding to either a positive or negative appraisal, (4) initiating available coping skills if the response is negative (e.g., helplessness, panic, anxiety, fear, confusion), and (5)

TABLE 6.5. Coping

- *Daily hassles:* those slight misfortunes that create ripples or interference in the flow of a day or week
- *Stressor:* any circumstance or object that is perceived as a potential threat to a person's physical, psychological, or social well-being
- *Coping:* the active and intentional use of cognitive and behavioral strategies to help mediate a stressful situation
- *Coping style:* a person's inclination to respond to a range of stressful situations in a particular way
- *Approach coping:* aiming coping attempts directly at the stressor
- *Avoidant coping:* directing strategies away from the stressor
- *Problem-focused coping:* attempts to change the stressor itself
- *Emotion-focused coping:* attempts to deal with the emotions related to the stressor
- *Coping strategy:* a response to a distressing situation that alters the situation or the person's perception of the situation so that it is no longer distressing
- *Cognitive appraisal:* process through which a person, guided by emotional responses to a situation, generates thoughts about, and makes meaning of, the situation
- *Self-care:* the intentional act of doing something that meets a self-need, not the needs of others

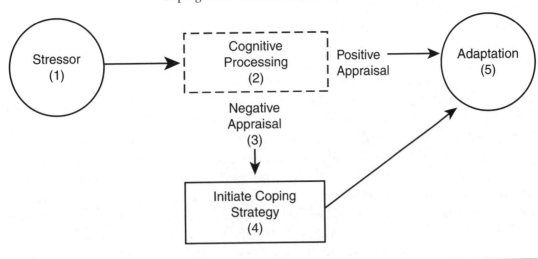

FIGURE 6.1. Stages of the coping experience.

adapting to the situation once the negative emotions diminish. As an illustrative example of the process, we describe the experience of a young child diagnosed with cancer in Figure 6.2. It is important to remember that individuals differ, and another child in this situation may have responded quite differently from Anna. It is difficult to predict a child's response to a particular situation or to judge the appropriateness of the response without knowing more about the stressor, the child, and the context within which the child is experiencing the stressor. However, the model presented above may guide us in predicting some aspects of a child's response.

Factors That Influence the Coping Process

Although we know that children make use of coping strategies when they feel threatened in some way, how or why a child chooses a particular coping strategy is a less clear. Researchers have identified a number of factors (beyond cognitive appraisal) that affect children's willingness and ability to initiate adaptive strategies to cope with stressors. Many models have been proposed to explain how specific intrapersonal, social, and environmental factors either facil-

Anna, an 11-year-old girl diagnosed with cancer, notices that the boy sitting next to her in math class has scribbled a caricature of her that exaggerates her least desirable physical features, including her hair loss [stressor]. Because of his popularity, she assumes that this view is shared by her classmates [Anna appraises the degree to which this situation threatens the stability she feels in her peer relationships]. As she tries to ignore him and continue her work [coping strategy], he leans toward her and says quietly, "What are you going to do, tell on me again?" [Anna appraises her capacity to deal with this comment.] She continues to focus on her assignment without saying a word to him [coping strategy]. Later that evening she becomes emotional as she describes the experience to her mother. She repeatedly says how much she "hates him" as she cries [coping strategy]. After a period of emotional expression, Anna calms down and brainstorms with her mother ways that she can respond the next time this happens [coping strategy].

FIGURE 6.2. Anna's coping experience.

itate or interfere with adaptive coping, thereby impacting a child's adaptation. The models also attempt to explain how each factor interacts with the others, how each affects a child's coping, and which factors have the most impact on coping.

One model, proposed by Wallander and Varni (1995), incorporates both risk and resilience factors to explain how one child may cope differently from another in a particular situation. The risk factors in this model are those stressors that make it more difficult for a child to adjust to his or her illness. Among these factors are the disease itself, teasing by friends, and family financial strain. Resilience factors, on the other hand, are those that may be helpful or protective for a child. The resilience component of the model is divided into three different categories: intrapersonal, sociological, and stress-processing factors. Intrapersonal factors may include the child's age, gender, degree of competence, attitude or temperament, and problem-solving ability. Family, peer, and school-based sources of support are examples of sociological factors. Stress-processing factors include cognitive appraisal and strategies (discussed earlier). A more thorough list of these factors is presented in Table 6.6.

Cognitive-behavioral models of coping with, and adjusting to, chronic illness often incorporate yet another component: the child or teenager's perceptions of the stressor and the availability of support (Moos, 2002). It is important to view the stressor from the student's perspective. Both perceived stress and perceived social support impact how a child copes with, and emotionally responds to, a stressor. A high level of perceived stress is often associated with negative emotional states (e.g., depression, anxiety), whereas perceived social support buffers the child from negative emotional states.

TABLE 6.6. Factors Influencing Coping

Disease and disability parameters
- Medical severity of illness
- Physical limitations
- Cognitive impairment
- Visibility of disease
- Chronic physical complications (e.g., diabetic neuropathy)
- Past trauma associated with hospitalization
- Functional independence (e.g., hygiene, self-management)

Intrapersonal factors
- Temperament
- Self-esteem
- Social assertiveness
- Optimism/positive outlook
- Problem-solving ability
- Age and developmental status
- Gender
- Sense of efficacy or mastery
- Perceptions of the disease (i.e., illness representations)
- Beliefs about treatment effectiveness

Social–ecological factors
- Family environment and supportiveness
- Social support resources
- Economic resources
- School involvement
- Friendships
- Teacher support

Stress-processing factors
- Cognitive appraisal
- Prior knowledge
- Attributions
- Child's perception of the situation (e.g., who is available to help, how threatening is the situation)
- Selection of specific coping strategies
- Coping style

Note. Parts of table adapted from Moos (2002) and Wallander and Varni (1995, 1998).

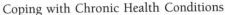

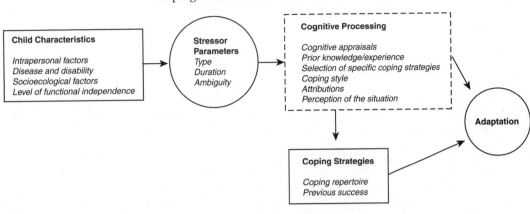

FIGURE 6.3. The coping experience—revised model.

As we incorporate information from these models into our "working" diagram, a more comprehensive view of the coping experience of chronically ill children emerges. Figure 6.3 presents the revised model. This model can be used as a tool to guide you in assessing, identifying, and designing appropriate interventions for students who are experiencing difficulty in coping with their condition in the school setting.

Assessment

You are likely to notice when children do not have adequate coping skills or when they are not using their coping resources to their fullest potential. Handout 6.3 (p. 130) presents a list of unhelpful coping skills that are often ineffective in the long term. There are several reasons why educators—you—play an important role in recognizing children who may need coping interventions. First, children spend a large portion of their waking hours in school, so you spend a lot of time with them and see much of their daily behavior. You are also able to observe children as they interact (or choose not to) with their peers and in various social situations. Finally, you are in a position to observe numerous aspects of children's development, such as their cognitive and physical abilities. Not only are you able to identify any deficits in these areas in comparison to other children, but you can also note any changes within a specific child over time. Children also trust their teachers, principals, and school counselors, so it is likely that you may be the person the child approaches and relies on when he or she needs help.

Because of this important role, it is very important for you to have the skills to assess children's coping behaviors in order to identify potential problems and prevent decline in functioning. We have developed a coping assessment worksheet, checklist, and student worksheet to facilitate this process of assessing a child's coping skills. Worksheet 6.1 (p. 99) is a checklist to be completed by school personnel; Worksheet 6.2 (p. 100) is a self-report instrument to be completed by the school-age child; and Worksheet 6.3 (p. 101) is a worksheet on which to compile the information gathered about the student, the problem, and the available resources. This information can then be used to develop interventions aimed at cultivating the student's use of more effective coping strategies.

Coping Interventions

Whereas children's coping styles are somewhat fixed, the coping strategies they use are generally easier to change. Coping strategies are specific learned behaviors that can be taught, modified, or altered to help the child meet his or her needs when managing a particular stressor. Our focus here is to help you learn how to work with children to change, learn, or enhance their coping strategies. Handout 6.4 (p. 131) describes several ways you can help support children during stressful times.

Cognitive-behavioral interventions have been shown to be very effective in helping children learn to cope more effectively with their illnesses. These interventions help children develop new skills and expand on those they already have, so that the additional stress of the illness does not become overwhelming for them. The focus of the cognitive-behavioral treatment differs depending on the specific needs of each child, but the general purpose is the same: to change the child's ineffective thinking and behaviors into effective ones. Three primary goals for helping children improve their coping strategies are: (1) teaching stress management, (2) enhancing social skills, and (3) increasing approach coping skills. Each of these goals is explained in greater detail below, and specific interventions are described later in this chapter.

Treatment Goals for Improving Coping

Stress Management

Stress management is a general term used to describe how a person negotiates stress in his or her life. Stress management skills may come more naturally for some children than others, just as some children are better at math or soccer. All children, no matter the skill level, can benefit from learning new multiplication strategies or practicing new soccer drills. Likewise, all children can benefit from learning new techniques or improving existing techniques for managing stress. Children with chronic illness or health conditions can learn a number of stress management techniques to help them cope. These may include learning to release tension, relax, or change the way they think about themselves and the illness. For example, a child may benefit from practicing guided imagery that allows him or her to relax during painful medical procedures or when he or she begins to feel anxious about going to the doctor's office. Relaxation and guided imagery exercises are helpful ways to teach the mind and body how to attain a state of calm and relaxation. Scientific studies have shown that relaxation has many benefits, including reducing stress, lowering blood pressure, and improving immune functioning (among other physiological and mental health benefits). Learning how to relax by using progressive muscle relaxation, passive relaxation, or guided imagery exercises is an easy and effective way to teach children to manage stress. When teaching each of the exercises below, be sure to find a quiet place where the child can relax and will not be disturbed. After the child gets into a comfortable position, guide him or her through the exercise by reading the scripts provided (or others that you find or create) aloud as the child follows your voice. It may be further helpful to record the exercise so that the child can practice at home.

Progressive Muscle Relaxation. Progressive muscle relaxation is an exercise designed to help the person experience the difference between the physical sensation of tension and relaxation in the body. Children are instructed to tense muscles, then relax them, and to pay attention to the difference in how their body feels. For example, a child would be told: "Now I want you to pretend that you have a big juicy lemon in one hand. I want you to try to get the juice out of that lemon by squeezing it as hard as you can for a few seconds. Go ahead. Make a fist and squeeze that lemon." After a few seconds the child would be instructed, "Now open your hand and let the drained lemon just drop to the floor." The instructor can then remind the child, "Notice the difference in how your hand felt when it was squeezing and how it feels now that it is relaxed, completely relaxed." This exercise is particularly helpful for those children who would benefit from becoming more aware of the signals their body is sending them, as well as children who do not believe they have control over their body (e.g., children with chronic headache or stomach pain, or those who are socially anxious because of their health condition). The child learns to pay attention to his or her body signals with the new awareness that it is possible to alter the sensations being experienced. Handouts 6.5 (p. 132) and 6.6 (p. 133) present progressive muscle relaxation scripts that can be used with children of all ages. We encourage you to use your own creativity to modify this script, so that it is more enjoyable for the child that you are helping.

Passive Relaxation. Like progressive relaxation, passive relaxation is particularly helpful for children who are highly anxious, worried, overwhelmed, or experiencing pain. Rather than asking children to physically tense and relax muscle groups, passive relaxation teaches them to pay attention to their breathing and their body as they imagine the tension, stress, or pain leaving the body, and feeling more and more relaxed as they do so. In this way, children learn to teach their body and mind to respond to verbal prompts to relax. With enough practice, they will be able to initiate a relaxation response during stressful situations. It is important for children who are taught relaxation exercises to practice them daily. Encourage them to practice whenever they have a few minutes of down time (e.g., riding home from school; just before bed). With practice, they will be able to induce relaxation more easily. Handout 6.7 (p. 135) presents a passive relaxation script that can be used with children of all ages. To facilitate the experience, first elicit some information about the problem they are experiencing and incorporate it into the script to make it more meaningful. For example, ask the children to give their pain a color (e.g., bright red) and to imagine their pain transforming into a color that is soothing to them, a color that is warm and relaxing (e.g., a soft white light).

Guided Imagery. Guided imagery is a third exercise that may help children to develop a coping skill by building on their natural ability to imagine. When the children are too young to understand the term "guided imagery," we refer to this exercise as "making pictures in their head." Children can use their imaginations to create (1) a safe place where they feel relaxed and pain free, (2) a helper (e.g., a person or creature) that can assist them when they are in need, or (3) a particular situation where they feel more in control.

Children who have difficulty talking about their difficulties or need a tool to help them escape during anxiety-generating situations (e.g., while injecting insulin or receiving a breathing treatment) will likely find benefits in learning guided imagery. Handout 6.8 (p. 136) presents an activity designed to help students learn guided imagery. Handout 6.9 (p. 137) presents a sample guided imagery script that can be adapted for children of all ages.

As you consider using these three stress management exercises, we again encourage you to be creative as well as to keep the script child focused. For example, a child will have more difficulty with the suggestion to "imagine your worries simply floating away" than with a more child-friendly suggestion such as "Imagine that there is an empty balloon on top of your head, waiting to be filled. Now let all the worries just escape through the top of your head and fill up this balloon. When the worries are gone, tie the balloon in your mind and let it drift up into the sky."

Stress management also involves helping students *change the way they think* about themselves, their illness, and the way others treat them. Helping children change unhelpful thoughts (e.g., about being "different") to more helpful thoughts (e.g., about being "special") can be particularly important for children with health conditions for whom bad things seem to outweigh good things in life. The exercises presented here are designed to help children who are stuck in negative thinking patterns to see that there are physical as well as emotional benefits to thinking more positively. Worksheet 6.4 (p. 103) is designed to help children identify healthy coping statements that they want to use to help reassure themselves when they feel stressed, worried, or overwhelmed. Worksheet 6.5 (p. 104) is intended to help children generate positive self-statements that will elicit positive emotions (e.g., relief, reassurance, comfort, hope) rather than the negative emotions that accompany their negative self-talk (e.g., anxiety, worry, depression). Worksheet 6.6 (p. 105) provides a structure for helping children change negative thoughts into positive ones that are more helpful. Finally, Worksheet 6.7 (p. 106) is an esteem-building activity that is designed to help children identify their personal strengths and recognize that these outweigh their limitations.

Social Skills

As discussed in previous chapters, children with chronic illnesses often struggle in their relationships with friends and family. Children may be teased for being different, may miss out on birthday parties because of their illness, or may be in conflict with siblings because of the attention their disease requires. Social skills training can be used to help children enhance their relationships and work through any problems that arise. Children might be given assertiveness training or taught how to deal with peer teasing. Here are a few guidelines: (1) Be sure you have a good understanding of what happened, (2) give the child several options for responding the next time teasing happens and ask him to choose, (3) have the child practice the responses, and (4) praise the child for practicing and using his new responses. (For more information on teasing, see the discussion in Chapter 4.)

Social skills training has been found to be especially effective with classmate relationships. For example, recruiting a positive peer to help a child reenter the school setting can make a big difference. Role playing may also be helpful because children can practice what to say if classmates tease or ask them about such things as having to take medicine in school. (Chapter 4 outlines actions that educators and parents can take to help children discuss their illness with peers, as well as how educators can help teach other students.) In addition, role playing can be used to help the other children develop and show their empathy for the child who is ill. The exercises in the following worksheets are designed to help children develop social skills that will be useful to them in their relationships. Worksheets 6.8 (p. 107) and 6.9 (p. 108) encourage children to problem solve and prepare to manage situations in which others are teasing them; Worksheet 6.10 (p. 109) encourages children to think ahead about the types of coping strategies they may use the next time they are feeling stressed; Worksheet 6.11 (p. 110) facilitates children's awareness of their support system; and Worksheets 6.12–6.14 (pp. 111–113) are designed to help children identify the issues that are causing them stress, practice using problem-solving skills, and normalize stress. Handout 6.10 (p. 139) provides students and educators with practical advice and guidelines for selection of peers to assist students with health conditions.

Approach Coping Skills

As discussed earlier in this chapter, children tend to function best when they use more approach, as opposed to avoidance, coping strategies. However, children may not always have these skills readily available to them, or they may have found that avoidant strategies have worked for them or others in immediate situations. After all, sometimes avoidance is desirable, such as when the child is experiencing temporarily painful procedures (e.g., shots). Cognitive-behavioral interventions can be designed to teach children how to actively approach the stressors related to their disease. This approach strategy may include helping children develop problem-solving techniques that could be used in deciding how to manage several areas: insulin treatments in school, changes in peer relationship, academic load, and so on. The following exercises are designed to facilitate an approach orientation to coping.

Feelings. Worksheet 6.15 (p. 114) is designed to assist students who have difficulty talking about, or identifying, the emotional aspects of stress. This activity is also an effective way to help peers develop a sense of empathy toward children who face unique health-related stressors.

Worksheet 6.16 (p. 115) is a journal page template. Children who have a hard time expressing their emotions verbally or in other healthy ways may find journaling particularly useful. (You might offer a child several copies so that he or she can create his or her own journal.)

Worksheet 6.17 (p. 116) can be used to help students (1) understand the connection between physical and emotional responses, (2) talk about their feelings, and (3) describe their pain or discomfort.

Worksheet 6.18 (p. 117) is a sentence completion worksheet in which a series of sentence stems is provided and the student is asked to complete each sentence. This exercise can provide a great deal of information about how the student is coping as well as allow the student to express problems that he or she may not be able to talk about directly.

Worksheet 6.19 (p. 118) can be used to facilitate a discussion with a child about the feelings that he or she does not express in public.

Grief. Worksheets 6.20 (p. 119) and 6.21 (p. 120) are designed to help children confront the grief that is naturally associated with chronic health problems. This activity helps them understand that it is okay to talk about the losses associated with their disease and to generate ideas about how they can mourn those losses.

Pain. Worksheets 6.22–6.24 (pp. 121–124) are designed to help students with pain understand what factors are involved in their pain and to assess their sensations or levels of pain. Pain can obviously interfere with children's ability to attend to, and benefit from, school activities. We have found these exercises to be very helpful in our work with children experiencing pain.

HELPING EDUCATORS COPE

Each day, educators work to fulfill the educational needs of children, including those with special needs. While you likely feel a sense of satisfaction from your work, it can also be demanding and stressful. Just like the children we have been discussing throughout this chapter, you too must cope with daily stresses, both related and unrelated to the children with whom you work. Working with children who have chronic health conditions may be a specific stressor for you in several ways, some of which are listed in Table 6.7.

Often in your desire to create a more stable, safe, and positive learning environment for students, it is easy to overlook your own needs. As an educator you must not only make it a priority to meet the needs of others, but also to recognize and care for your own personal needs. It is impossible to help others if you do not first take care of yourself. Developing positive self-care practices will help you improve the quality of your work, enhance your own physical health, and act as a buffer against the threat of burnout that is

---

TABLE 6.7. Stressors for Educators Working with Ill Children

- Added workload
- Witnessing child's suffering
- Experiencing loss
- Feeling responsible for the child
- Anxiety about your own children
- Fear of medical emergencies
- Uncertainty of parents' or employers' expectations

often associated with excessive levels of stress. In addition, you will be serving as a role model for the children by taking care of your own physical and emotional health.

Self-care is *the intentional act of doing something that meets one of your needs, not the needs of others.* It is about taking care of yourself in all dimensions of your life—body, mind, and spirit. Self-care is not just something you need to employ during times of crisis; rather, it is something that should be integrated into your daily life. Only when we are healthy and our own physical and emotional needs are met can we provide the best support and nurturing possible to meet the needs of children. Are you taking care of yourself? Take these brief self-assessments and find out.

Worksheet 6.25 (p. 125) is an activity designed to help you identify the physical, cognitive, emotional, and spiritual signals that you are being given regarding your own needs for self-care. After you review the list and identify the signals that your body, mind, and spirit are giving you, take a moment to think of an activity that would promote self-care in each of the areas that you marked. Put this list somewhere visible so that you can be reminded of your self-care needs daily.

Common Myths about Self-Care

The following are a few of the common misconceptions many of us hold about self-care. Often these are the kinds of beliefs that keep us from doing what we need to do most—which is to take care of ourselves so that we can do our work more effectively.

• *Myth 1. Taking care of your own needs is selfish.* This belief is a common self-care myth. We assume that taking care of ourselves means that we will have less time to meet the daily demands that surround us, including demands from administration, community, family, parents, and students. However, experts point out that when we take care ourselves, the quality of our lives and relationships improves and our productivity increases. We are actually able to be of greater service to others when we are taking care of our own well-being. We understand that we can make the choice and do not need to feel either guilty or selfish when we put our own needs and well-being first.

• *Myth 2. Needing self-care is a sign that you are weak.* Many of us assume that people who engage in self-care activities only do so because they cannot handle stress or manage the daily demands of their lives. We might see them as immature, fragile, or weak. However, self-care serves to replenish and strengthen you not only when you are feeling run down, but also when you are feeling good, to maintain this sense of well-being.

• *Myth 3. Self-care takes too much time and money.* Self-care does not require a large time commitment. Spending as little as 15 minutes each day can really make a difference. It is not necessary to spend a lot of money on expensive services (e.g., traveling, therapy, massage) or materials (e.g., books, workout equipment, new clothes) in order to adequately take care of yourself. Many self-care activities do not cost a dime. It is possible to find activities that help you to relax and rejuvenate regardless of your income or place of residence. Handout 6.11 (p. 140) reframes these myths, reminding you that self-care is not only good for you but it is something you owe yourself and the children you wish to help.

What Happens When We Neglect Our Own Needs?

When we do not take care of our own needs, it becomes more difficult to recognize and address the needs of others, including those of students. Neglecting self-care may have a negative impact on our work, health, and life, in general. Some of the consequences of neglecting our own self-care are listed in Handout 6.12 (p. 141).

Sometimes, even when we do take care of ourselves, the stress in our lives may be too much to handle on our own. Often, sharing our feelings and concerns can be very helpful, even if that simply means discussing them with friends, family members, or colleagues. Many professionals who work with individuals with health conditions reach a point at which they choose to seek professional help themselves. Seeking counseling is another form of self-care that may be especially helpful when stress begins to interfere with your daily functioning. If you begin to feel overwhelmed by feelings of depression, anxiety, or any of the other signs indicated on the checklist for assessing your own self-care needs, it may be beneficial to find a professional service to help you deal with your own life stressors. This help may come in the form of individual counseling, a support group, or Internet resources.

How Can We Increase Our Daily Coping Capacity?

There are several steps we can take to care for ourselves on a regular basis, whether or not we are showing signs of stress. Self-care works best as a method of preventing stress, so using self-care techniques is important even when we do not necessarily feel stressed. It is more obviously important when we notice ourselves showing or feeling many of the signs on the checklist for assessing self-care needs. Worksheet 6.26 (p. 127) introduces a list of activities that we have found to be positive methods of self-care. Highlight or circle those that appeal to you. Place this list in a location where you will see it each morning, so that you can select one activity to do for yourself that day. As you review the list, take note of other self-care ideas that come to mind.

CONCLUDING COMMENTS

Throughout this chapter we have discussed the significant role educators play in identifying children who are not coping well and helping them develop more effective ways of managing both the common and the health-related stressors in their lives. At this point you should feel familiar with the coping terminology, understand the flow of the coping process, and have a greater awareness of the factors that may potentially influence a child's coping. Additionally, we remind you of the critical nature of attending to your own self-care needs as the first step toward helping students. A number of worksheets are provided that you may feel free to use or modify for use with the children you support. With the information and these tools in hand, we hope that you can view your role as a unique opportunity to make a difference in the lives of your students.

WORKSHEET 6.1. Assessment of Student's Coping

Directions: The checklist below is divided into four areas in which a student may have difficulty coping. Place a checkmark next to each term or phrase that describes the student's behavior in the past *2 weeks*. Checkmarks may indicate areas in which the student may require intervention to help expand coping skills. It is important not to mark statements as true if they are solely caused by the physical limitations of the student's illness.

General stress:

_____ Grades have dropped

_____ Easily irritated

_____ Worries about things a lot

_____ Seems sad, down, or blue

_____ Gets angry easily and/or often

_____ Tires or fatigues easily

_____ Difficulty concentrating

_____ Fails to complete homework

_____ Argues often (with peers, teachers, etc.)

_____ Restless or fidgety

Pain:

_____ Winces or grimaces, indicating pain

_____ Withdraws from physical education or recess

_____ Struggles with, or refuses to engage in, activities that do not seem physically demanding (e.g., writing, playing an instrument)

Doing treatments:

_____ Often "forgets" medicine or treatment

_____ Leaves treatments/medicines at home frequently

_____ Minimizes symptoms of importance (e.g., denies pain to be allowed to play kickball)

Social/peer relationships:

_____ Withdrawn, does not interact with peers

_____ Teased by other students or teases other students

_____ Plays alone or wants to stay with the teacher at recess or lunch

_____ Speaks in class only rarely or never

WORKSHEET 6.2. My Coping Toolbox: An Assessment of Student's Coping

Name: _____ Date: _____

Directions: No two people cope with a situation in exactly the same way. We all use a different set of tools to deal with things that give us stress or make us worry. Below is a list of "skills" or "tools" that you might use when you need to deal with stress. We would like to know which of these tools are in your toolbox. Put a check next to the tools that you have used *in a 2-week period* when you were dealing with a difficult or stressful situation.

When dealing with stress, I:

☐ Write about it for myself.

☐ Write to someone about it.

☐ Talk to a teacher or counselor.

☐ Talk to my brother or sister.

☐ Pray about it.

☐ Take a nap or sleep.

☐ Say positive things to myself.

☐ Talk to my pet.

☐ Watch TV or a movie.

☐ Talk to my friend.

☐ Cry.

☐ Think of all the things I can do to help.

☐ Act silly.

☐ Don't give up.

☐ Talk with a coach.

☐ Tell myself I can handle it.

☐ Do something I like (a hobby).

☐ Take a walk or a bike ride.

☐ Run or exercise.

☐ Sing.

☐ Play a sport with someone else.

☐ Relax; try to be less tense.

☐ Read a book.

☐ Try to fix the problems.

☐ Ask friends for help.

☐ Focus on finding a way to handle it.

☐ Listen to music.

☐ Scribble or draw something.

☐ Ask someone I respect for advice.

☐ Practice the things I learned to do to help.

WORKSHEET 6.3. Coping Assessment Worksheet

1. **Student information**

    Student's name:_____   Teacher: _____

    Age: _____   Grade: _____

2. **Relevant history**

    Provide brief relevant academic, family, medical, psychosocial, behavioral, social, and cultural history.

3. **Reasons for assessment**

    A. List behavioral, emotional, social, academic concerns here and, when appropriate, identify the source(s) of information (e.g., "Ms. Miller, the librarian, reported that Jane seems to be isolating herself from her classmates during library group time"):

    B. List specific problems in any of the following areas.

    Eating _____

    Medication or treatment _____

    Health concerns _____

    Peers _____

    Physical activities _____

    Relationships _____

    School _____

    C. Describe the details and context within which the identified problem(s) is occurring:

(continued)

4. **Coping analysis**

   A. Assessment of current coping

   Briefly summarize findings from assessments, observations, and information obtained from interviews or other sources.

   B. Initial hypothesis

   Hypothesize about the possible reasons for the apparent obstacles to effective coping.

5. **Problem solution**

   List potential interventions that appear to be appropriate for the identified problems.

6. **Evaluation**

   List tools or methods that might be useful for monitoring intervention progress and evaluating intervention outcome.

Completed by: _____   Date: _____

WORKSHEET 6.4. Coping Statements

Did you know that you can change the way you feel about something by changing the way you talk to yourself about it? *Coping statements* are helpful words you say to yourself when you are stressed, worried, or overwhelmed so that you feel better.

Directions: Below is a list of coping statements. Circle the statements that you want to use.

I am a good person.

I have friends I can trust.

I will feel better soon.

I am good at some things.

People love me and take care of me.

I am a survivor.

I like the way I look.

I'm good at lots of things.

I can handle this situation.

I will not let them get me down.

I can handle this.

Things will get better.

I know it hurts now, but I will feel better soon.

I can still do most of the things I want to do.

I can take good care of myself.

I know I can do it.

I feel relaxed.

I feel good right now.

The doctors are helping me feel better.

WORKSHEET 6.5. My Self-Talk

Self-talk is what you say to yourself, and sometimes other people, about yourself. Self-talk affects how you feel. When you talk negatively to yourself, your feelings will probably be negative, too. For example, when you say, "I will never feel better," you may begin to feel sad or angry.

Directions: Below are some examples of self-talk statements that kids say to themselves. Fill in a *Smiley Face* next to the self-talk statements that are positive and a *Frowney Face* next to the negative statements.

◯ "I will never feel better. My pain will never go away."

◯ "I can help myself feel better by taking a couple of deep breaths when I feel tense."

◯ "I always feel so tired. Will this feeling ever end?"

◯ "When I start to feel bad, I can close my eyes and go to my favorite place in my mind. When I do this, I notice that I start to feel better and I have control over how I feel."

You have the power to change your negative self-talk statements to positive ones!

My Negative Statement

◯

_____
_____
_____

My Positive Statement

◯

_____
_____
_____

Did you know that what you think affects how you feel? Worrying or thinking negatively can make the good things about yourself hard to find. What worrying, angry, or negative thoughts do you have?

Directions: In the jagged shape below, write a negative thought or worry. Below the shape, draw a picture of you. What do you look like on the outside when you are having this negative thought or worry on the inside? Then, in the cloud, find a way to CHANGE and rewrite the negative thought or worry into something more positive. Again draw a picture of you. What do you look like on the outside when you are having this positive thought on the inside?

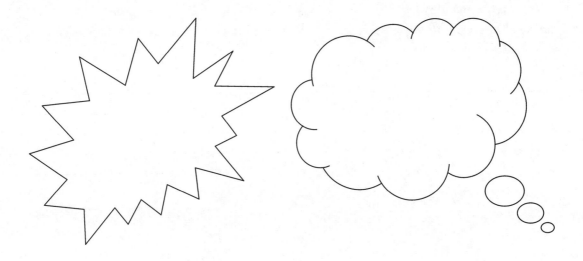

Negative thought or worry   Positive thought

WORKSHEET 6.7. Building Self-Esteem

Do you know what it means to have self-esteem? Self-esteem is the way you see and think about yourself. The more positive things you see, think about, and know about yourself, the better your self-esteem and the better you feel. Did you know that you could change your self-esteem simply by changing the way you think about yourself?

Directions: On the lines below, make a STRENGTHS list (the things you are good at or like about yourself) that is longer (heavier) than your LIMITATIONS (the things you're not so good at or are unable to do) list. When you cannot think of any more, ask your parents, friends, teacher, or coach for help with thinking of more strengths.

My Strengths	**My Limitations**
Example: *"I'm good with numbers. Math is easy for me."*	Example: *"I have a hard time talking."*

WORKSHEET 6.8. Tease Buster Worksheet

Though everyone gets teased some of the time, and though teasing can be done in the spirit of friendship, it can also be just plain mean. When it's hurtful, here is what I think is going on:

People tease when they get a response . . . it makes them feel more powerful, and that's their reward. Teasing back doesn't do much good. In fact, it usually just brings you down to the same level as the teaser, and nothing positive gets accomplished. So, take away the reward by taking away the response that teasers learn to expect. Here's what I've found to be helpful:

- Try not to be drawn into the teasing.
- When it starts, make a joke of it or respond with a comment that you've practiced at home, or walk away while casually saying "Well, I'm out of here . . . better things to do to have fun" without appearing hurt. In other words, develop what's called "resilience."
- Think of yourself as a rubber ball instead of a glass that can be shattered easily.

Teasing also happens when people are uncomfortable or scared. If you're being teased because of a difference that others don't understand, how about helping them?

- Assume that they wouldn't tease if they knew more about the difference. You're the expert on it; you're the one who's learned how to live with it; so you're the one in the best position to teach them about it.
- Here's an example. Say your hair came out during treatment to get rid of cancer. That happens to a lot to kids, and it's confusing and scary to children who don't understand. So there you are, with your baseball cap on, walking into the cafeteria at school. Who should you meet but the biggest bully in school, who pushes your cap to the ground and says, "Ooh, baldy, what happened, cooties eat your hair?" You might say, "Nope, you got that one wrong! I'm taking some strong medicine that my hair just didn't like, so it took off for awhile. I wonder what color it'll be when it grows back . . . "

Directions: In the boxes below, write the things that kids say to you that are hurtful. Then write at least one idea on how you could respond to that statement the next time it happens.

The silly things people say	Tease busters (how I want to respond)

WORKSHEET 6.9. The Little Giraffe: Social Skills Exercise

Goals:

- Help the child identify feelings about peer teasing.
- Enhance problem-solving skills in social situations.

Materials:

- Story
- Stuffed animals

Description:

Begin this exercise by reading the story to the child, prompting the child at the indicated times. (Match the giraffe's gender with the child's.) After the story, engage the child in a problem-solving discussion about what the giraffe could do in this situation. Allow the child to use the stuffed animals to act out what the giraffe could do, if he or she desires. Then help the child recreate the story or tell a different story with a more positive and adaptive ending.

The Little Giraffe

Once upon a time there was a little giraffe named _____. He [she] was a bright and special giraffe. One day the little giraffe wanted to play a game, but none of the other giraffes would play with him [her]. The other giraffes always called him [her] names like _____ because he [she] was a very special giraffe and wasn't like all the others. Being called mean names made the little giraffe feel _____. Sometimes being special made him [her] feel very _____, but on days like today, it made him [her] feel _____. Often the little giraffe would try to say something when the other giraffes teased him [her], but usually he [she] was too _____. Sometimes he [she] would be feel so upset that he [she] would cry. Even though the little giraffe tried not to let the teasing bother him [her], sometimes he [she] just couldn't stop those negative feelings. What could the little giraffe do to help himself [herself] in this situation? Are there people that might be able to help the little giraffe? What are some things that the little giraffe could say to the other giraffes?

WORKSHEET 6.10. What Can I Do?

Everyone has good days and bad days. Sometimes the bad days seem like they last forever. Some kids have found that when they don't feel good or they are having a bad day, it helps to plan what they can do to help them through a hard time.

Directions: Below is a list of activities that other young people your age have used to help them. Circle at least *three ideas* that you will try the next time you are having a hard time. Then share this list with your parents or teacher so they have a better idea of how to best help you.

Write about it for myself (keep a diary).

Talk with someone about it.

Pray about it.

Try to fix the problem.

Talk to my friend.

Watch TV or a movie.

Take a walk or a bike ride.

Tell myself I can handle it.

Cry.

Do something I like (a hobby or activity).

Sing.

Play a sport with someone.

Read a book.

Focus on the best way to handle it.

Scribble or draw something.

Write to someone about it (a letter).

Create calming pictures in my mind to relax.

Say positive things to myself.

Talk to my pet.

Spend time with my best friend.

Run or exercise.

Practice the thing I've learned to do to help.

Act silly.

Don't give up.

Relax my body.

Ask a friend for help.

Listen to music.

Think of all the things I can do to help myself feel better.

Ask someone for advice.

Other things that I do: _____

_____

_____

It may be helpful to share this list with your parents or teacher
so that they can give you the help you need.

WORKSHEET 6.11. Building a Circle of Support

Everyone needs help from other people sometimes (kids and adults!). Sometimes we know who is in our Circle of Support and sometimes we have to remind ourselves who we can turn to when we need to ask for help. This activity will help you to figure out who you can go to if you need help with troubles you may have with your schoolwork, with friends, with your illness, or anything else.

Directions:
Part I. List the names of the people that are there to help you when you need them.

_____

_____

_____

Part II. Now write your name in the circle below and draw a larger circle around it. Write the names of the people you feel the most comfortable asking for help and would go to first if you needed help. Then draw a larger circle around this one and write the names of the people who you would go to if none of the people in the first circle were able to help you. Now draw a larger circle around these and write the names of the people you know that you do not really feel very comfortable asking for help. You just created your own reminder of your Circle of Support.

Part III. List the circumstances or situations that might lead you to ask for help and use your circle of support.

_____

_____

_____

WORKSHEET 6.12. Carrying a Lot on My Shoulders

Directions: Everyone (kids and adults!) experiences stress. This activity is designed to help you to remember this and to identify what brings you "stress."

Part I. List as many problems or worries as you can think of that other people you know experience. (Remember: *All* people experience stress or worry!)

_____

_____

_____

_____

Part II. You will need an 8 × 10 piece of white paper, a few pieces of colored paper, tape, and markers or crayons to complete this activity. First, cut out, or ask an adult to cut out, 10 pieces of colored paper. Write a different problem or worry that you have on each. Next, draw a picture of yourself. Be sure to include *only* your head and shoulders on the page. Tape each "problem" or "worry" onto the self-portrait, stacking them on each shoulder. See how much you carry on your shoulders.

Part III. With an adult to help you, think about how you can solve each problem or cope with each worry on your picture. When you find a way to cope with a problem or worry, you can remove it from your picture, and if you want, crumple it up and throw it in the garbage.

Everyone feels worried or stressed at times, especially when we carry too much on our shoulders. When this happens, it is important to talk to someone else about our problems and try to find ways to cope with each problem or worry (one at a time!), so that we feel better.

Counselor Notes:

WORKSHEET 6.13. Look Back

Situations do not always go the way we may want them to. But no need to worry, you can learn something from every situation, even those that do not go well, if you take time to *look back*. You have the chance to look back on a situation and figure out how you would do it differently if it happens again. Follow these five easy steps:

1. Close your eyes and imagine the situation in your mind. Rewind the picture in your mind to the beginning of the situation. As you play it back, look closely. What is happening? Who is there? Pay attention to what you are doing and saying.

2. Open your eyes and tell the story about what happened. Write it, draw it in a series of pictures, or say the story into a tape recorder. Be sure to talk about the key events that happened in order. For example, if you write it, start with: When I look back at what happened, I see. . . . If I could do it again, I would do it differently. Here is my new plan. . . .

3. Read, look at, or listen to the story. If something went well, write it down and circle or underline what you wrote. Write down or put a box around the things that did not go well.

4. Now think about what you would change if this happens again. How could you respond differently? Write, draw, or record your new plan on tape.

5. Give the plan a title—make sure it is one that will help you to remember it when you need it!

Signed: _____ Date: _____

WORKSHEET 6.14. My Body Knows

Directions: To complete this activity you will need scissors, glue sticks, paper, and crayons or markers.

Part I. Body's Talk

Bodies have different ways of reacting to worries or problems. These "reactions" are our body's way of telling us that we feel worried, anxious, nervous, or scared. For example, when some people feel nervous, their hands may shake. Other people start to sweat or their mouth might get really dry. Some people feel like they have "butterflies" in their stomach if they are worried, scared, or nervous.

Part II. My Body
Using colored paper, cut out shapes that represent "reactions." For example, you could cut paper into the shape of rocks to represent a feeling of "heaviness," a sun to represent a feeling of "sweating" or "warmth," and butterflies to represent "funny feelings" in your stomach.

Now draw an outline of your body (you can make it life size if you have paper that is long enough!). Inside the lines, glue the "reactions" to the places on your body where you feel each of them when you feel worried or upset. For example, if you feel "heaviness" on your shoulders, glue the rocks on top of your shoulders. If you feel "butterflies" in your stomach, glue a few butterflies near your stomach.

Part III. Listening to My Body

Finally, find an adult to talk with about the picture you created. Explain how this picture represents what your body knows and how your body communicates to you when you are feeling worried, anxious, nervous, or scared. Talk about each cutout and the thoughts or events that make your body feel that way. Then talk about what you could do to cope when you feel worried, nervous, or scared. Who or what could help you with this worry or problem?

Signed: _____   Date: _____

WORKSHEET 6.15. How Would You Feel?

Directions: For each situation listed on this worksheet, describe the feeling you would probably have if it happened to you. Also, think about why you think you might feel that way.

Situation	Feeling
Your friends make fun of you because you have to go to the nurse's office every day after lunch.	
When you look in the mirror, you do not recognize yourself.	
Someone asks you, "Why do you look so funny?"	
Your parents tell you that you can't play your favorite sport anymore.	
You always get picked last to play on a team.	
Other kids think you have cooties or that they can catch your illness.	
You're afraid you will never feel better.	
Your doctor told you that you may only eat the food that is on the list he gave you. The list does not include any of your favorite foods.	
When you are in the hospital, your classmates send you get-well cards.	
You have 40 days of homework to make up because you missed 2 months of school.	
Your friend sticks up for you when kids tease you.	
You can't play your favorite game or activity at recess anymore (e.g., jungle gym, dodge ball).	

WORKSHEET 6.16. My Personal Journal

Name: _____   Today's date: _____

Some of the **THOUGHTS** I had during the past week about myself, my family, school, or other things were . . .

_____

_____

_____

_____

Some of the **FEELINGS** I felt during the past week were (circle the feelings) . . .

Happy	Sad	Excited	Lonely
Curious	Scared	Worried	Proud
Mad	Tired	Bored	Thankful

Write other feelings here: _____

_____

Some of the **ACTIVITIES OR THINGS** I did this past week were . . .

_____

_____

_____

_____

Some of the **OTHER THINGS** that were important about this past week are . . .

_____

_____

_____

_____

WORKSHEET 6.17. Color Your World

Directions: Sometimes we feel our feelings in our bodies. Draw a picture of yourself below and color in any of the feelings you feel using the colors listed. You may feel certain colors in certain parts of your body (e.g., you may feel afraid in your stomach). You can color in certain parts of your body or anywhere you like.

Sad = Blue

Afraid = Black

Guilty = Brown

Angry = Red

Jealous = Green

Nervous = Orange

Happy = Yellow

Lonely = Purple

Excited = Pink

WORKSHEET 6.18. About My Feelings

I feel afraid when . . .
I feel disappointed when . . .
I am really good at . . .
I am ashamed of . . .
I get excited when . . .
I feel frustrated when . . .
Most of the time I feel . . .
I am happy when . . .
I feel upset when . . .
I am sad when . . .
I am calm when . . .
I was really mad when . . .
I am thankful for . . .
I am lonely when . . .
I hope that . . .

WORKSHEET 6.19. Masks

Directions: Sometimes people try to hide how they are feeling from other people. Using the circles below draw faces that show the feelings you sometimes hide from others.

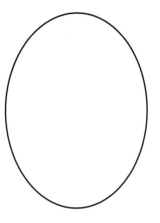 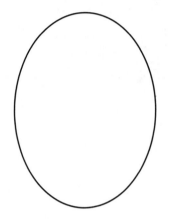 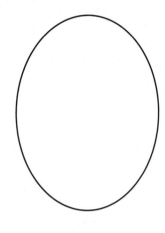

_____   _____   _____

Now draw faces that you use to hide the feelings you drew above.

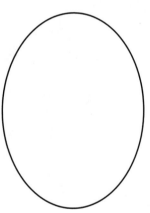 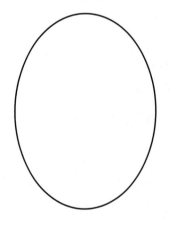 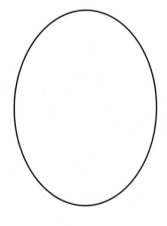

_____   _____   _____

WORKSHEET 6.20. Grief

Getting sick or feeling pain can bring many feelings. The sadness or anger that is felt because of the losses and changes is called GRIEF. Some kids we know have found this list of ideas helpful when they are feeling grief.

- Talk about how you feel with your parents.

- Call a close friend.

- Write about how you feel in a journal or on the computer.

- Send a letter or e-mail to a friend about your grief.

- Let yourself cry.

- Find someone to hug.

- Read and learn more about grief.

- Talk to your teacher or coach or school counselor.

- Find a friend to whom you feel close.

- Create a picture of your grief with paint, crayons, or markers.

- Make a collage with pictures that represents your grief.

- Take a walk with your pet and talk about how you feel.

- Make something meaningful out of clay.

- Play with friends.

- Write a poem.

Directions: List the ideas that would be helpful to you.

_____

_____

_____

WORKSHEET 6.21. Losses

Children's lives change when they are diagnosed with a chronic illness. You may have lost some things that are important to you. Here is what some kids have told us about their losses.

I can't run as fast as I used to before I got sick.—Zach, 10 years old

I lost my good grades. Schoolwork seems harder to me.—Jenny, 14 years old

I lost my hair during my cancer treatment.—Chris, 11 years old

Directions: On the lines below, write about things important to you that you have lost because of your health condition.

_____

_____

_____

_____

_____

_____

_____

WORKSHEET 6.22. The Pain Puzzle

WHAT IS THE PAIN PUZZLE?

Scientists are trying to figure out how pain works and what can be done to make pain better. So far, pain is still a puzzle to be solved. We are starting to solve the pain puzzle. We do know that how we feel, what we think, and what we and other people do about our pain can make that pain better or worse.

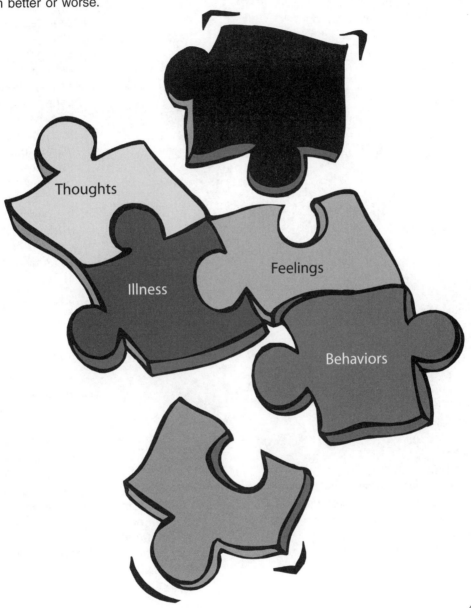

(continued)

PAIN PUZZLE DESCRIPTION

Thoughts

Thoughts can make pain worse, like "I can't stand this pain. I will never feel any better." But helpful thoughts make pain better, like "I don't like this pain, but I can stand it. I just need to do some things to make my pain better."

Feelings

Feelings such as being worried, sad, or angry can make pain worse. You might worry that your pain is getting worse, or you may get angry because it stops you from doing some fun things. You might also get discouraged and feel sad because your pain keeps you from feeling good and doing what you want. More positive feelings can make pain get better. You might be happy that the pain will go away or glad that you can do something to help the pain.

Illness

This is what happens in your body when you have pain. There are many pain fibers that pick up signals when something bad happens, like when you get hurt. The signals are carried up to your brain and back down again. These signals can be changed by other parts of the pain puzzle to make the pain feel better.

Behaviors

What you do when you are in pain is important. When you hurt, you might ask for medicine, rest, or move more slowly. These behaviors let others know, like your parents, doctor, or teacher, that you hurt or are in pain so they can help you. You want to try to stay as active as you can, even when you hurt. You may need to change how you do things to keep from hurting as much.

WORKSHEET 6.23. Connect the Puzzle Pieces

Which piece of the pain puzzle goes with each of the statements below? Draw a line from each statement in the left column to the name of the puzzle piece in the right column.

I'm sad that it hurts to play.

THOUGHTS

I don't want to do anything but sit and watch TV.

ILLNESS

This pain is bad, but I know that it will be over soon.

FEELINGS

This pain is bad, and I don't think I can stand it.

I think I need to rest.

BEHAVIORS

It hurts when I run.

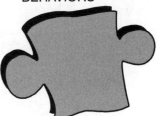

WORKSHEET 6.24. How I Feel

Your name _____ Today's date is _____

1. Put a mark on the line that best shows *how you feel now.*

|—————————————————|—————————————————|

I feel no pain or hurt.　　　I feel some pain or hurt.　　　I feel the most pain or
　　　　　　　　　　　　　　　　　　　　　　　　　　　　　　hurt possible.

2. Color red *lightly* where you get *little* aches and pain.

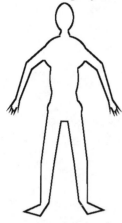

Color *bright* red where you get *BIG* aches and pains.

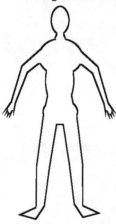

3. Put a mark on the line to show what was the *worst pain you had this week.*

|—————————————————|—————————————————|

I feel no pain or hurt.　　　I feel some pain or hurt.　　　I feel the most pain or
　　　　　　　　　　　　　　　　　　　　　　　　　　　　　　hurt possible.

WORKSHEET 6.25. Checklist for Assessing Your Own Need for Self-Care

Your body, mind, and spirit will signal you when you neglect your own needs. This activity is designed to help you identify the messages that you are being given regarding your own needs for self-care.

Directions: Review the following list and check those signs that are true for you. This checklist should help you see the areas of your life that may need some extra attention or self-care. Examine the items that you mark carefully. Next to each checked item, write a self-care activity that will help you attend to this signal.

SIGNALS

REMEDIAL ACTIVITY

Body signs

Body self-care

____ I am frequently bothered by aches and pains.

_____

____ I typically do not feel well rested.

_____

____ I am easily frustrated or irritable with others.

_____

____ I have difficulty falling or staying asleep.

_____

____ I have headaches and/or stomach problems.

_____

____ I have problems with my hearing.

_____

____ I often feel my heart pounding.

_____

____ I have rapid, shallow breathing.

_____

____ I often feel weak or dizzy.

_____

____ I no longer engage in activities that used to give me pleasure.

Mental signs

Mental self-care

____ I often feel confused or have disorganized thoughts.

_____

____ I have difficulty making decisions.

_____

____ I have difficulty problem solving.

_____

____ I have memory problems or am often forgetful.

_____

____ I have difficulty concentrating or paying attention.

_____

____ I have many negative thoughts or worries.

_____

____ I have difficulty communicating my thoughts.

_____

____ I frequently have bad dreams or nightmares.

(continued)

SIGNALS   REMEDIAL ACTIVITY

Behavioral signs   **Behavioral self-care**

____ I am often reluctant to leave my home or bed.   _____

____ I have withdrawn from friends and family.   _____

____ I neglect good nutrition and/or exercise.   _____

____ I participate in fewer enjoyable activities.   _____

____ I am less interested in sex.   _____

____ I have increased my use of drugs and/or alcohol.   _____

____ I cry frequently or am easily brought to tears.   _____

____ I am easily startled by small sounds.

Emotional signs   **Emotional self-care**

____ I feel sad or blue.   _____

____ I feel guilty.   _____

____ I am often angry, even for no particular reason.   _____

____ I feel helpless and/or hopeless.   _____

____ I feel burned out or worn out at the end of the day. _____

____ My mood shifts rapidly.   _____

____ I am often unable to feel emotions.

Spiritual signs   **Spiritual self-care**

____ I feel angry at a higher power.   _____

____ I have withdrawn from my spiritual or religious community.   _____

____ I pray or meditate less frequently.   _____

____ I lack an interest in expressing my spirituality.   _____

WORKSHEET 6.26. Examples of Self-Care Activities

- Meditate.
- Pray.
- Practice yoga.
- Practice breathing and relaxation techniques.
- Step outside and get some fresh air.
- Talk to someone about your troubles (friend, coworker).
- Spend time with family and friends.
- Talk to your pet.
- Spend time with others in your spiritual/religious community.
- Establish a "buddy system" with your coworkers.
- Go to bed early.
- Take a day off.
- Stay home when you are physically sick.
- Get enough sleep.
- Take a nap.

- Take a walk.
- Play a sport.
- Jog.
- Play with children.
- Dance.
- Play a game.
- Sit under a tree.
- Sit by the water.
- Forgive someone.
- Tell a joke.
- Share funny stories.
- Laugh as loud as you can.
- Do something silly.
- Make someone else laugh.
- Think about something for which you are grateful.

- Help someone in need.
- Avoid criticizing others.
- Say something good about yourself.
- Find a hobby.
- Sing a song.
- Feel the wind on your face.
- Silently watch a sunset with a friend.
- Watch the clouds.
- Sit in the sunshine.
- Dance in the rain.
- Watch children play.
- Write down your thoughts and feelings.
- Cry when you need to.
- Look at old photos.

List other activities that are enjoyable to you.

_____

_____

_____

_____

_____

_____

_____

HANDOUT 6.1. How to Help a Child with Health Concerns

- Help the student with medical treatments or medication routines.

- Support the student in peer relationships and social activities.

- Model healthy ways of coping with difficult situations.

- Help the student make up missed assignments or lessons.

- Assist in developing an accommodation or intervention to help the student meet his or her optimal potential.

- Monitor the student's health and well-being.

- Provide positive feedback to the student and his or her parents.

- Acknowledge the student's strengths and communicate these to him or her as well as the other educators.

- Design specific interventions to help the student cope during the school day.

HANDOUT 6.2. Developmental Differences in Coping

Infancy and toddlerhood

During this early period of development, children generally have very little understanding of their illness. Because of their newly emerging but limited verbal skills, they often must use other means of communicating their needs to adults. During this period children are beginning to develop a sense of trust and an overall sense of security. Illness-related experiences such as pain, hospitalization, invasive treatments, and restriction of motion may create new challenges for children and potentially interfere with the development of their sense of trust, safety, and security.

Preschool

For children ages 3–5, the desire and need for autonomy becomes increasingly important. Preschoolers may understand that they are sick, but they may not understand what caused their symptoms or illness. For example, a 4-year-old boy may believe that throwing up causes him to get sick, rather than the fact that he is throwing up because he is ill. Because of preschoolers' movement toward independence, hospital stays and rigorous medication schedules can feel as if they are challenging the children's natural desire to do more by themselves. Preschoolers may counter this lack of control over their world by challenging the limits set by the adults around them. Adults can help by allowing children the choices that they can make but working with them to complete aspects of the treatment that must be done. For example, the child might be asked if she wants to take the pink pill first or the white pill or to take her pill before or after lunch. Taking the pill is not the option, but how it is done can be a choice-filled experience for the child.

Early school age

Children in the first few years of elementary school continue to work toward developing a sense of mastery over their environment. In this phase, children are aware of, and can articulate, reasons for their illness, although these reasons may not seem to make sense to the adults around them. During this time, children engage in what has been called "magical thinking," in which they believe that they are the cause of events. For example, a child may believe he caused the illness because he lied to his parents, called his teacher a name, or did not eat his vegetables. The illness also begins to effect peer relationships because children this age have more awareness of how they are different from their peers. Adults can help by reassuring them that the illness is not their fault, help them learn more about how their body works, and provide opportunities for them to help in managing their illness when possible (with close adult supervision, of course).

Older school age

Children this age are better able to understand their illness and its treatment. Although some children this age appear quite mature at times, adults should not assume that children's understanding and responses should be similar to their own. Children's strong desire and need to belong may be threatened if they feel left out when absent from school or social activities with their peers. Protecting ill children by restricting them from activities with other children may be done in their best interest, but adults must realize the distress this creates for them. Such restrictions can interfere with children's independence and sense of mastery. When possible, adults can help ill children to stay involved on some level and participate in whatever way they can.

Adolescence

During the teenage years the development of a personal identity separate from family is beginning to emerge. The importance of appearance and self-image increases, which, of course, can create difficulties when medication or treatment results in changes in appearance, such as loss of hair, bloating, or weight gain. With their increasing sense of independence, it is not uncommon for teens to go through times of denial of their illness. This denial may be observed when a teen neglects to take medications, follow special diets, or check blood sugars. Additionally, there are natural physiological changes that are also occurring during this period that can, at times, lead to symptom changes or changes in medication dosages. Adults can best help teens by supportively encouraging them to manage their disease. Remember, teens living with a chronic illness are still teens! It is important to talk about teen issues, such as independence, college planning, dating, sexuality, and substance abuse.

HANDOUT 6.3. Unhelpful Coping Strategies

Everyone uses both helpful and unhelpful coping strategies at times. This is especially true for students who may not have the experience to develop many helpful strategies. When you notice students using unhelpful strategies, such as those listed below, recognize that they are attempting to deal with their stress, but may need help finding new, more helpful ways to do so.

- Giving up or quitting
- Acting out/disrupting
- Acting bossy
- Trying to control others
- Pretending stress isn't a problem
- Making excuses
- Cheating
- Trying to get attention using destructive means
- Lying

HANDOUT 6.4. Methods of Supporting Students Experiencing Stress

- See the student as a person, not as his or her illness.
- Accept the child.
- Model healthy ways to cope.
- Educate yourself about the child's illness and treatment.
- Play an active role in supporting the child.
- Answer questions from the child as well as other students.
- Coordinate your support efforts with the child's parents and health care team.
- Develop a plan for handling medical emergencies.
- Help the child think positively.
- Know the mandatory and optional tasks in the child's routine.
- Identify difficulties in the child's social life and work with the child to create solutions.
- Help the child understand his or her illness better.
- Be available to listen.
- Make accommodations for the child's limitations.
- Always look for a child's strengths and be sure to acknowledge those strengths to the child.
- Take care of yourself to ensure that you can help others.

HANDOUT 6.5. Three Steps to Relaxation: A Scripted Introduction
to Progressive Muscle Relaxation

Directions to child: Find a quiet place where you will not be disturbed to practice these exercises. Get your body into a comfortable position before we begin.

STEP 1: Relaxation

When you are hurting, tense, or worried, you might notice that your muscles feel tense or tight. This exercise will teach you how to relax so that you feel more positive and can keep your mind off your pain and stress. To do this, you will learn how to breathe deeply and how to tense and relax your muscle groups.

Squeeze this tennis ball in your hand and then relax your grip. Now try it again. Tense and relax. Notice the difference between the tension and the relaxation? Put down the ball and, while lying down, try tensing your other muscles just like you did with the tennis ball.

First tense your ARMS and HANDS. And now relax them. Try it again. Squeeze and relax.
First tense your FACE and NECK. And now relax them. Try it again. Squeeze and relax.
First tense your STOMACH and BACK. And now relax them. Try it again. Squeeze and relax.
First tense your LEGS and FEET. And now relax them. Try it again. Squeeze and relax.

STEP 2: Deep breathing

Deep breathing is something you can do anywhere! When you focus on your breath, your body becomes more relaxed and your mind is not thinking so much about your pain and stress.

1. Start by breathing slowly in through your nose (if you can!). Keep your shoulders relaxed (try hard not to raise them up to your ears!).
2. Place you hand on your belly. Try to expand your belly and chest outward. It should feel like your belly is blowing up like a balloon.
3. Slowly let your big breath out through your mouth, like you are blowing out a candle.
4. Now start again!

Try to take 10 breaths this way. Whenever you get the chance, PRACTICE . . . just before bed, waiting in line, sitting in class, walking down the hallway, any time, any place!

STEP 3: Now let's put them together!

Breathe in slowly, and as you breathe in . . . tense your ARMS and HANDS.
Breathe out slowly, and as you breathe out . . . relax your ARMS and HANDS.
Breathe in slowly and as you breathe in . . . tense your FACE and NECK.
Breathe out slowly, and as you breathe out . . . relax your FACE and NECK.
Breathe in slowly and as you breathe in . . . tense your STOMACH and BACK.
Breathe out slowly, and as you breathe out . . . relax your STOMACH and BACK.
Breathe in slowly and as you breathe in . . . tense your LEGS and FEET.
Breathe out slowly, and as you breathe out . . . relax your LEGS and FEET.

HANDOUT 6.6. Scripted Progressive Muscle Relaxation for Children

Today we're going to practice some special kinds of exercises called *relaxation exercises*. These exercises will help you to learn how to relax when you're feeling uptight and help you get rid of those butterflies-in-your-stomach kinds of feelings. They're also kind of neat, because you can learn how to do some of them without anyone really noticing. In order for you to get the best feelings from these exercises, there are some rules you must follow. First, listen to what I say and try to follow along, even if it seems kind of silly. Second, you must focus and do what I say. Third, you must pay attention to your body throughout these exercises, pay attention to how your muscles feel when they are tight and when they are loose and relaxed. And fourth, you must practice. The more you practice, the more relaxed you can get. Do you have any questions? Are you ready to begin? Okay, first, get as comfortable as you can in your chair. Sit back, place both feet on the floor, and just let your arms hang loose. That's fine. Now close your eyes and don't open them until I say to. Remember to follow my instructions very carefully, focus, and pay attention to your body. Here we go.

Hands and Arms

Pretend you have a whole lemon in your left hand. Now squeeze it hard. Try to squeeze all the juice out. Feel the tightness in your hand and arm as you squeeze. Now drop the lemon. Notice how your muscles feel when they are relaxed. Take another lemon and squeeze. Try to squeeze this one harder than you did the first one. That's right, real hard. Now drop the lemon and relax. See how much better your hand and arm feel when they are relaxed. Once again, take a lemon in your left hand and squeeze all the juice out. Don't leave a single drop. Squeeze hard. Good. Now relax and let the lemon fall from your hand. [Repeat the process for the right hand and arm.]

Arms and Shoulders

Pretend you are a furry, lazy cat. You want to stretch. Stretch your arms out in front of you. Raise them up high over your head. Pull them back, way back. Feel the pull in your shoulders. Stretch higher. Now just let your arms drop back to your side. Okay, kitten, let's stretch again. Stretch your arms out in front of you. Raise them over your head. Pull them back, way back. Pull hard. Now let them drop quickly. Good. Notice how your shoulders feel more relaxed. This time let's have a great big stretch. Try to touch the ceiling. Stretch your arms way out in front of you. Raise them way up high over your head. Push them back, way back. Notice the tension and pull in your arms and shoulders. Hold tight now. Great. Let them drop very quickly and notice how it feels good and warm and lazy.

Jaw

Imagine you have a giant jawbreaker bubble gum in your mouth. It's very hard to chew. Bite down on it hard! Let your neck muscles help you. Now relax. Just let your jaw hang loose. Notice how good it feels just to let your jaw drop. Okay, let's tackle that jawbreaker again now. Bite down hard! Try to squeeze it out between your teeth. That's good. You're really tearing that gum up. Now relax again. Just let your jaw drop off your face. It feels good just to let go and not have to fight that bubble gum. Okay, one more time. We're really going to tear it up this time. Bite down as hard as you can. Harder. Oh, you're really working hard. Good. Now relax. Try to relax your whole body. You've beaten that bubble gum. Let yourself go as loose as you can.

Face and Nose

Here comes a pesky old fly. He has landed on your nose. Try to get him off without using your hands. That's right, wrinkle up your nose. Make as many wrinkles in your nose as you can. Scrunch up your nose real hard. Good. You've chased him away. Now you can relax your nose. Oops, here he comes back

(continued)

again, right back in the middle of your nose. Wrinkle up your nose again. Shoo him off. Wrinkle it up hard. Hold it just as tight as you can. Okay, he flew away. You can relax your face. Notice that when you scrunch up your nose, your cheeks and your mouth and your forehead and your eyes all help you, and they get tight too. So when you relax your nose, your whole body relaxes too, and that feels good. This time that old fly has come back, but this time he's on your forehead. Make lots of wrinkles. Try to catch him between all those wrinkles. Hold tight now. Okay, you can let go. He's gone for good. Now you can just relax. Let your face go smooth, no wrinkles anywhere. Your face feels nice and smooth and relaxed.

Introduction

Stomach

Hey! Here comes a cute baby elephant. But he's not watching where he's going. He doesn't see you lying in the grass, and he's about to step on your stomach. Don't move. You don't have time to get out of the way. Just get ready for him. Make your stomach very hard. Tighten up your stomach muscles real tight. Hold tight. It looks like he is going the other way. You can relax now. Let your stomach go soft. Let it be as relaxed as you can. That feels so much better. Oops, he's coming this way again. Get ready. Tighten up your stomach real hard. If he steps on you when your stomach is hard, it won't hurt. Make your stomach into a rock. Okay, he's moving away again. You can relax now. Kind of settle down, get comfortable, and relax. Notice the difference between a tight stomach and a relaxed one. That's how we want to feel—nice and loose and relaxed. You won't believe this, but this time he's coming your way and there's no turning around. He is headed straight for you. Tighten up. Tighten hard. Here he comes. This is really it. You've got to hold on tight. He's stepping on you. He's stepped over you. Now he's gone for good. You can relax completely. You're safe. Everything is okay, and you can feel nice and relaxed.

This time imagine that you want to squeeze through a narrow fence and the boards have splinters on them. You'll have to make yourself very skinny if you're going to make it through. Suck your stomach in. Try to squeeze it up against your backbone. Try to be as skinny as you can. You've got to be skinny now. Just relax now and feel your stomach all warm and loose. Okay, let's try to get through that fence again. Squeeze up your stomach. Make it touch your backbone. Get it real small and tight. Get it as skinny as you can. Hold tight now. You've got to squeeze through. You got through that narrow little fence with no splinters! You can relax now. Settle back and let your stomach come back out where it belongs. You can feel really good now. You've done fine.

Legs and Feet

Now pretend that you are standing barefoot in a big, fat mud puddle. Squish your toes down deep into the mud. Try to get your feet down to the bottom of the mud puddle. You'll probably need your legs to help you push. Push down, spread your toes apart, feel the mud squish up between your toes. Now step out of the mud puddle. Relax your feet, let your toes go loose, and feel how nice it feels to be relaxed. Now go back into the mud puddle. Squish your toes down. Let your leg muscles help push your feet down. Push your feet hard. Try to squeeze that puddle dry. Okay. Come back out now. Relax your feet, relax your legs, relax your toes. It feels so good to be relaxed. No tenseness anywhere. You feel kind of warm and tingly.

Conclusion

Stay as relaxed as you can. Let your whole body go limp and feel all your muscles relaxed. In a few minutes I will ask you to open your eyes, and that will be the end of this practice session. As you go through the day, remember how good it feels to be relaxed. Sometimes you have to make yourself tighter before you can be relaxed, just as we did in these exercises. Practice these exercises every day to get more and more relaxed. A good time to practice is at night, after you have gone to bed and the lights are out and you won't be disturbed. It will help you get to sleep. Then, when you are really a good relaxer, you can help yourself relax at school. Just remember the elephant, or the jaw breaker, or the mud puddle, and you can do our exercises and nobody will know. Today is a good day, and you are ready to feel very relaxed. You've worked hard, and it feels good to work hard. Very slowly, now, open your eyes and wiggle your muscles around a little. Very good. You've done a good job. You're going to be a super relaxer.

HANDOUT 6.7. Scripted Passive Muscle Relaxation for Children

Rationale: This exercise is designed to help children relax. It may work best to record an adult's voice, or have the child record her voice, reading the script so the child does not have to focus on the script while relaxing. Another option is to have someone read the script to the child. The script should be read in a calm, flowing manner. The child should be allowed to get comfortable and close her eyes if she desires.

Script

Begin by letting your mind drift . . . just letting any thoughts float away, not paying attention to any one thought for a long period of time. Begin to pay attention to your breathing, noticing each breath you take—in and out, just noticing your breathing, in and out.

Now pay attention to your arm. You may notice that your arm is feeling warm . . . and heavy [*pause*]. You may feel the warmth through your arm, and the heaviness of your arm . . . your arm feeling warm and heavy, relaxing a little more and noticing the warmth drift across your body and into your other arm.

Now pay attention to your other arm. You may notice that your arm is feeling warm . . . and heavy [*pause*]. You may feel the warmth through your arm, and the heaviness of your arm . . . your arm feeling warm and heavy, relaxing a little more, noticing that both arms are feeling warm and heavy and both arms are feeling more and more relaxed. And that warm, heavy relaxation begins to drift . . . from your arms, down through your tummy, and into your leg.

Now pay attention to your leg. You may notice that your leg is feeling warm . . . and heavy [*pause*]. You may feel the warmth through your leg, and the heaviness of your leg . . . your leg feeling warm and heavy, relaxing a little more and noticing the warmth drift across your body and into your other leg.

Now pay attention to your other leg. You may notice that this leg is feeling warm . . . and heavy [*pause*]. You may feel the warmth through your leg, and the heaviness of your leg . . . your leg feeling warm and heavy, relaxing a little more and noticing the warmth throughout both legs . . . both legs feeling warm, feeling heavy, feeling more . . . and more . . . relaxed.

Now notice that the warmth in your legs and arms is spreading over your whole body . . . spilling out across your feet . . . your hands . . . your neck and shoulders . . . your face and head. Warm and heavy . . . your whole body feeling warm and heavy and relaxed.

Now it's time to slowly come back out of this position, still feeling relaxed and calm. Whenever you are ready, you may open your eyes . . . wiggle your toes and fingers a little . . . move your arms and legs a little . . . move your head and neck. And whenever you're ready, you can move around, but still feeling relaxed and calm.

HANDOUT 6.8. Pictures in Your Head: A Script for Guided Imagery

Directions: Find a quiet location where you will not be disturbed to practice these exercises. Close your eyes and use your imagination to think of your favorite ice cream. Can you see it in your mind? What does it look like? What color is it? Is there whip cream on top? Can you feel how cold it is? Some of the images you can create in your mind are helpful and fun, others are not. When you are hurting or feeling down, you might have images that you don't like or that bother you. To help you feel better, we are going to practice changing the pictures in your head into something more helpful.

"Peaceful Places" Practice Exercise

Close your eyes and practice imagining in your mind's eye that you are at each of the places noted below. Once you have the image, look around and tell me what you see. Listen carefully and tell me what you hear. Take time to notice the fragrances and tell me what you smell. Try to touch something in the image and tell me what you feel.

A BEACH   A LAKE   YOUR FAVORITE PLACE

THE MOUNTAINS   A MEADOW

"Untying the Knots" Practice Exercise

If there is some aspect of your disease that you have an ugly or negative picture of, let's change that into something different. For example, close your eyes and picture your painful joints feeling as if a rope were tied tightly around those painful areas. Now picture the rope beginning to loosen its knot, and soon the knot is so loose that it just becomes very limp; just like your joints, limp and relaxed. Now picture your red hot joints turning cool blue. Now you try it. Write down a description of your ugly or negative pictures. Have someone help you change your painful picture into a picture that is more helpful. Then close your eyes, imaging a more helpful picture, and know that it will always be there when you need it!

HANDOUT 6.9. Scripted Imagery Exercise for Young Children

Directions to teacher: Find a quiet location where you will not be disturbed and read this as the child uses his or her imagination.

Script

Once upon a time there was a young man named Chris. He was an amazing child. Chris liked playing with other kids and wrestling with his dog, named Leo. He liked making people laugh, and he would make funny faces and noises just to hear their laughter. He also liked making up new games with his friends, playing outside, and taking care of his pet fish. Of course, Chris was like other kids in lots of way, but he always felt a little different. Chris was a creative child. One of his favorite things to do was to make up stories. See, Chris thought that stories were the best way to feel better when things weren't going the way he wished that they would. Sometimes he felt lonely, like when it was time to go to bed. Sometimes he got frustrated, like when his friends didn't come over to play. Sometimes he got scared, like when he was in the hospital and he had to have special tests. And sometimes he was just plain bored, like when there was nothing fun to do. Lucky for Chris he had a special gift—the gift to create stories or picture in his head. And guess what? You do, too. As you listen, Chris will teach you how to do this and tell you when you might want to use this special gift.

First, pay close attention to how your body feels. Just by concentrating on your body, you can make your body feel real loose—loose like a bowl of jello or loose like a rag doll. Here's how to do it. Take very, very slow breaths in through your nose and blow out through your mouth, and with every single breath, feel your body getting more and more relaxed. Relax even more until it almost feels like your body is floating on a cloud. Get a picture of the cloud in your head and see yourself riding on the cloud. Now shake your hands as fast as you can as I count out loud to five. Don't they feel tingly? Next stretch your arms way up to the sky while you take a giant breath, a giant breath of bright blue sky that is all around you. Fill yourself up with this clean, fresh air. Now pretend that your fingers are bringing some of the calm air from the sky back down to your tummy, and while your fingers come back down from the sky, gently blow out the air that you saved inside your lungs. Doesn't the air feel good? It feels good to me because it tickles my tummy and reminds me that I can use my special gifts to go wherever I want to go, and to be whatever I want to be.

Now it's time to close your eyes very gently and pretend that you are walking on a beach. As you walk, notice what is around you. Look up into the sky and find the sun. Perhaps the big beautiful sun is behind the clouds for now. As the sun peaks through the clouds, you can feel the rays of light sun shining down on you. It's very warm, and as you feel the sun, it makes you feel warm, safe, and comfortable. As you walk on the beach, notice how your body feels. It's not too hot. It's not too cold. In fact, it is just about right. Now find a place to sit down in the sand near the water. As you sit, stretch your legs and let your toes touch the water. Feel the tiny little waves touch your feet. Feel the wet water on your feet. Then watch the waves go back into the ocean. The water feels so cool on your skin. Smell the air, too. As you sit here, you may remember another time that you were at the beach. Perhaps you were with your family or friends. Sometimes paying attention to the smells of the beach is a good way to remember special times. Notice if you can sense any fragrances. Now look out into the water and see that there is a sailboat. It's out there in the ocean, and the waves make it bob up and down, down and up, in the gentle, blue water. The sun is shining down on the boat and on the beach where you are now lying down relaxing. Imagine that this boat is a bright shiny green color, with big white sails. Just see how beautiful the boat is. Look at its size and its shape. Notice if there are any people in the boat and if you know any of them.

(continued)

Now, look over and find a large box of crayons in the sand right there next to you, crayons with brand new pointy tops and lots of bright colors. Choose your very favorite color, and use your magic to draw a daydream in the sky or in the sand. Draw anything you like. Once I drew a silly purple snake with a great big smile and long black eyelashes, because I was lonely and I wanted a friend. And guess what? It helped me to not feel so lonely. Draw whatever you like. Take 2 minutes, which is all the time you will need to draw something that might help you feel better right now [*pause for 2 minutes*].

Now, put the box of crayons back in the sand next to you. Stand up with both feet in the sand and again let the water run over your feet. As you feel the warmth of the sun, turn back and begin walking the way you came, knowing that this beach will be here waiting for you the next time you wish to return. This is your special place and you can return to it any time you need by just picturing it in your mind. As you walk, listen to my voice as I count backwards from 5 to 1. With each number you will begin to feel more and more awake. *Five* (5), you are feeling yourself awaken with each step. *Four* (4), you're feeling more energy in your body as you continue to move forward, closer to my voice. *Three* (3), halfway to feeling completely awake. *Two* (2), feeling more and more rested and awake as you leave the beach and come back into this room. *One* (1), you are completely awake and back into this room. You can open your eyes when you are ready.

HANDOUT 6.10. Positive Peers

Sometimes students need help adjusting socially to their chronic illness. Some may need help when returning from an extended school absence or hospitalization. Others may struggle with a particular part of their social adjustment and development. In either case, it may be helpful to find a positive peer to help the young person cope with some of the difficult social demands he or she faces. One of the most important parts of a positive peer system is choosing appropriate students to serve as the peers. Here are a few guidelines to help you with this selection process.

A positive peer should:

- Be similar in age to the student he or she will help
- Be socially comfortable and knowledgeable
- Be knowledgeable, or willing to become so, about the student's health condition
- Be willing to allow the student to enter into his or her own social group, or be willing to engage with other groups to help him or her do likewise.
- Be willing to communicate regularly with the teacher and, possibly, the parents.

Once the positive peer has been chosen, both the student's and the potential peer's parents should be consulted. Parents can help develop goals and make suggestions to the peer to help facilitate the process. After everyone has been introduced to the idea and has agreed to the positive peer system, the positive peers can begin to help facilitate the student's social development and adjustment in the following ways.

- Model healthy coping skills and positive friendship skills.
- Model appropriate social interaction in groups and later talk to the student about the interaction; if it seems appropriate, provide suggestions about the interaction.
- Be supportive if the student you are helping is nervous or uncomfortable in certain social situation; do not make fun of or embarrass him or her.
- Talk to your teacher and the student's parents about how things are going or if you have concerns.
- Just simply be a good friend.

HANDOUT 6.11. Dispelling the Myths of Self-Care

- Taking care of your own needs is NOT selfish. It is a necessary step if you desire to help others.

- Needing self-care is NOT a sign that you are weak. It is a sign of self-compassion.

- Self-care does NOT take a lot of time and money. The best forms of self-care are free and can be accessed anytime, anywhere.

HANDOUT 6.12. The Consequences of Neglecting Self-Care

When you neglect self-care, you may . . .

- Feel less productive at work

- Have less energy

- Feel less motivated

- Be more likely to get physically sick

- Need more frequent medical care

- Experience difficulty in relationships

- Become more pessimistic or cynical

- Experience less pleasure and satisfaction in your life

- Be more vulnerable to stress, anxiety, and depression

7

Tying It All Together

with JAMI GROSS *and* RAELYNN MALONEY

Over the course of this book, you have learned about the educational, social, emotional, and physical needs of children with chronic health conditions. You have learned about the conditions themselves and how they may affect a child in an educational setting. You have also learned about accommodations for children with chronic illness and how to develop and integrate plans that provide those accommodations. We have addressed integration and reintegration issues in detail. Finally, we have talked at length about children's coping and how to help both them and yourself cope more effectively. We have designed this chapter to help integrate all of the hands-on information from previous chapters.

In the first section we use a case example to demonstrate the tools we have discussed. In the second section we provide information about a model program as well as two Web-based resources that have been established to help children with chronic illnesses and their families adjust to their conditions, as well as to help educators in their work with this group. We have compiled a list of Internet and published resources if you wish to locate more information about various issues related to children with chronic illnesses. The specific objectives of this chapter are:

- To use a case example to discuss reentry, accommodations, social issues, and coping in children with chronic health conditions.
- To provide information about three specific resources available to help children, parents, and professionals deal with a child's chronic illness.
- To provide various other resources you can access if you want more information about children's health issues and coping.

CASE EXAMPLE: ELISA

In this section, we discuss the case initially presented in Chapter 1, outlining the school-based assessments and interventions implemented to help Elisa function better and succeed in the school setting. We cover her reentry, the accommodations made, as well as the processes of assessing and aiding Elisa in her coping. We use the worksheets and other tools provided throughout this book to illustrate each piece of this process, just as we hope you will do, using this book as a resource. For the purposes of illustration, we utilize many more worksheets than would be typically used in the case of a single student.

Background Information

Elisa is a 12-year-old Caucasian girl of Latin descent who has been receiving treatment for cancer. She has been absent from school for nearly 2 months, recently returning to attend school for half-days. She is often sleepy, irritable, and fatigued while in school, and she often cries and asks to go home. Her parents are firm in their decision to keep her in school for half-days. Elisa's parents also prefer to maintain as much privacy as possible regarding the course and prognosis of her treatment.

Reentry Plan

An Illustration of the Process

Elisa has been back in school attending half-days for 1 month. Now that she has successfully completed her medical treatments, her parents would like to see her fully integrated back into the classroom. They are asking that she begin attending full time by the beginning of March 15 (approximately 6 weeks from today). With this timeline in mind, use the outline provided in Chapter 5 (p. 77) to help you develop an integrated reentry plan prior to Elisa's return to assist with her transition back to school. Figure 7.1 is an illustration of what Elisa's reentry plan might look like. Remember, it is important that this plan reflect a collaborative effort between the school, Elisa, Elisa's parents, and her health care team.

What Educators Need to Know about Elisa

As Elisa returns to school, there are several pieces of information that educators will need in order to best help everyone involved—Elisa, her parents, teachers, peers, and administration. Chapter 2 provides a general overview of childhood cancer that would be a good start to understanding some of the issues that may arise with Elisa's reentry into school. The resources provided later in this chapter may be beneficial as well. However, Elisa's parents and physicians, as well as Elisa herself, are likely to be the best informants regarding her disease and related needs. Implementing a successful reentry plan, which allows for contact with the doctors and nurses involved in Elisa's care, can facilitate the gathering of the necessary information. Figure 7.2 provides an outline of the type of information you may need to know about Elisa's health condition. Some of the questions in this figure are addressed more thoroughly by tools demonstrated later in this chapter.

Student's Name: Elisa R. Smith

Expected date of completion	Plan of action	Implementer
Week 1	1. Identify a school liaison as the primary contact for Elisa's family and medical team.	Principal
	2. Communicate with Elisa's health care team regarding school reentry.	School Liaison (e.g., School RN)
Week 2	3. Obtain materials regarding Elisa's illness to be provided to teachers and other appropriate school personnel.	School Liaison
	4. Schedule achievement and other tests to assess cognitive functioning, if appropriate.	School Liaison
Week 3	5. Conduct needed assessments.	School Psychologist
	6. Meet with a member of the health care team to discuss relevant information about Elisa's academic performance and educational needs.	Teacher
	7. Obtain contact information (e.g., names and telephone numbers) of Elisa's treating physician and a contact person at the clinic/office.	School Liaison/Teacher
Week 4	8. Begin to prepare Elisa and her classmates for reentry.	Teacher/Counselor
Week 5	9. Invite or request that a member of the health care team (with Elisa, if she chooses) make a presentation to help answer students' questions.	School Liaison/Teacher
	10. Continue to process any issues, concerns, and questions with students prior to Elisa's return.	Teacher/Counselor
Week 6	11. Maintain contact with the health care team and parents to provide ongoing assessment of Elisa's adjustment	School Liaison/ Counselor

FIGURE 7.1. Sample school reentry plan for Elisa.

Assessing Elisa's Level of Functioning and Participation

It is very important, for multiple reasons, to assess Elisa's level of functioning. First, if you assume that Elisa is functioning at the same level she demonstrated prior to cancer and treatment, she may become frustrated with herself, you, and the school. It is possible that work is more difficult or that she tires more easily now. Thus, maintaining the same expectations you may hold for her peers or that you may have held for Elisa prior to cancer, could cause significant problems in her readjustment to school. On the other hand, if you assume that Elisa cannot do certain activities or tasks because of her recent illness, she may feel bored or unhappy that people think of her differently. This misunderstanding, too, may hinder Elisa's adjustment and coping. Therefore, it is important to gain a thorough understanding of her physical, emotional, and cognitive resources as she reenters school. It is also important to assess her functioning repeatedly, as it may change during different stages of the reentry process. Figure 7.3 (adapted from Table 4.3) and the assessment worksheets (see Figures 7.4, 7.5, and 7.6) may be used to assess Elisa's functioning at any point during the reentry process. Table 5.5 in Chapter 5 (pp. 69–71) also provides

1. What kind of cancer does Elisa have? <u>Leukemia</u>

2. What is her prognosis? <u>Would rather keep private.</u>

3. What treatment has Elisa received/is Elisa receiving now? <u>She had chemo and may have further</u> <u>treatment in the future.</u>

4. What side effects might Elisa experience from her treatments? <u>She lost her hair.</u>

5. Does Elisa have any physical limitations? <u>Tires easily; has to wear mask in public.</u>

6. What does Elisa know about her disease? What does she call it? <u>She knows about it and calls it</u> <u>"cancer," not Leukemia.</u>

7. What can I tell Elisa's peers and teachers about her disease? <u>Would like to tell them as little as possible</u> <u>about Elisa, but it might be nice to have a cancer specialist come in to meet with her class.</u>

8. Does Elisa have any medical appointments coming up? <u>She will have several follow-up appointments</u> <u>in the coming months.</u>

FIGURE 7.2. Informational needs of educators: What to ask parents and medical professionals about Elisa's health.

Date: <u>January 1, 2003</u>   Next Assessment Needed: <u>March 2003</u>

Assessment Completed by: <u>Mr. Hope</u>

	Level 1: Mild	Level 2: Mild to moderate	Level 3: Moderate	Level 4: Severe
Is the child handicapped?	No	Possibly	Yes	Yes
How does it affect the child's functioning?	Health impairment does not interfere with day-to-day functioning and learning.	Health impairment does not interfere with learning, but there is a possibility of unusual episodes or crises.	Health impairment either presents frequent crises, or else so limits the child's opportunity to participate in activities that it interferes with learning.	Health impairment is so severe that special medical attention is regularly needed. The child's opportunity for activity is so limited that he or she may not be able to participate in a regular classroom.
Must the program be modified?	No	No change in program planning is necessary. Be aware of the potential for unusual occurrences. Report them to the parents or doctor. Know any first-aid procedures that might be required.	Activities will have to be modified to allow a health-impaired child to participate. Staff must know proper first-aid procedures and be prepared to deal with children's questions about crises.	Extensive staff and program alterations are necessary to accept child into program. Home- or hospital-based programs may be more appropriate. Classroom support from medical services will be necessary, if child is in classroom.

FIGURE 7.3. Sample assessment of level of functioning and program modifications for Elisa.

Directions: The checklist below is divided into four areas in which a student may have difficulty coping. Place a checkmark next to each term or phrase that describes the student's behavior in the past *2 weeks*. Checkmarks may indicate areas in which the student may require intervention to help expand coping skills. It is important not to mark statements as true if they are solely caused by the physical limitations of the student's illness.

General stress:

_____ Grades have dropped

__X__ Easily irritated

_____ Worries about things a lot

__X__ Seems sad, down, or blue

_____ Gets angry easily and/or often

__X__ Tires or fatigues easily

__X__ Difficulty concentrating

_____ Fails to complete homework

_____ Argues often (with peers, teachers, etc.)

_____ Restless or fidgety

Pain:

__X__ Winces or grimaces, indicating pain

__X__ Withdraws from physical education or recess

_____ Struggles with, or refuses to engage in, activities that do not seem physically demanding (e.g., writing, playing an instrument)

Doing treatments:

_____ Often "forgets" medicine or treatment

_____ Leaves treatments/medicines at home frequently

__X__ Minimizes symptoms of importance (e.g., denies pain to be allowed to play kickball)

Social/peer relationships:

__X__ Withdrawn, does not interact with peers

_____ Teased by other students or teases other students

__X__ Plays alone or wants to stay with the teacher at recess or lunch

_____ Speaks in class only rarely or never

FIGURE 7.4. Sample assessment of student's coping.

information about medical conditions and their impact on sports participation—another piece of important information that may be useful in evaluating Elisa's overall functioning.

Accommodations for Elisa

Because of the physical, cognitive, emotional, and behavioral impact that Elisa's illness and treatment are likely to have, it may be necessary to provide her with specific accommodations to facilitate her successful readjustment to school. The basis of these accommodations will need to come from several sources. First, Elisa and her parents will likely be able to provide some information about how Elisa's illness has affected the way her brain and body work. It is possible that a pediatric psychologist at the hospital tested Elisa before

Name: _Elisa Smith_   Date: _1/3/03_

Directions: No two people cope with a situation in exactly the same way. We all use a different set of tools to deal with things that give us stress or make us worry. Below is a list of "skills" or "tools" that you might use when you need to deal with stress. We would like to know which of these tools are in your toolbox. Put a check next to the tools that you have used _in a 2-week period_ when you were dealing with a difficult or stressful situation.

When dealing with stress, I:

☑ Write about it for myself.   ☐ Tell myself I can handle it.

☐ Write to someone about it.   ☐ Do something I like (a hobby).

☐ Talk to a teacher or counselor.   ☐ Take a walk or a bike ride.

☐ Talk to my brother or sister.   ☐ Run or exercise.

☐ Pray about it.   ☐ Sing.

☑ Take a nap or sleep.   ☐ Play a sport with someone else.

☐ Say positive things to myself.   ☐ Relax; try to be less tense.

☐ Talk to my pet.   ☐ Read a book.

☐ Watch TV or a movie.   ☐ Try to fix the problems.

☐ Talk to my friend.   ☐ Ask friends for help.

☐ Cry.   ☐ Focus on finding a way to handle it.

☐ Think of all the things I can do to help.   ☑ Listen to music.

☐ Act silly.   ☐ Scribble or draw something.

☐ Don't give up.   ☐ Ask someone I respect for advice.

☐ Talk with a coach.   ☐ Practice the things I learned to do to help.

FIGURE 7.5. Sample of My Coping Toolbox: An Assessment of Elisa's Coping.

and after her treatment to assess whether any changes occurred. Find out if this testing was done and if you can obtain any information about the assessment. Finally, Elisa's teachers, parents, and health professionals should be able to provide some information about any changes they have observed since her return. All of this information should be used together to complete an accommodations checklist like the one found in Figure 7.7.

Elisa's 504 Plan

It is possible that Elisa's illness and treatment have affected her to such an extent that a 504 plan should be implemented. Chapter 4 outlines the rationale for 504 plans, as well as how they differ from individualized education plans. Figure 7.8 contains an example of a 504 plan that could be designed to help Elisa when she returns to school.

Disclosure about Elisa's Illness

One of the most difficult issues for families is often what and how to tell others about a child's illness. Elisa's parents have indicated that they would like to keep much of Elisa's health-related information private. However, they realize that the school personnel and peers will need to be told something about Elisa's absence and current status in school.

1. **Student information**

   Student's name: <u>Elisa Smith</u>   Teacher: <u>Ms. Robinson</u>

   Age: <u>12</u>   Grade: <u>7th</u>

2. **Relevant history**

   Provide brief relevant academic, family, medical, psychosocial, behavioral, social, and cultural history.

   Elisa is a 12-year-old Caucasian girl of Latin descent. Although her parents divorced when Elisa was in 3rd grade, both continue to be active and involved parents. Elisa has a younger sister who is in elementary school. In November of last year Elisa was diagnosed with cancer, for which she subsequently was hospitalized and underwent treatment. Prior to diagnosis and treatment, Elisa performed in the high-average range academically. She was involved in several extracurricular activities, including cheerleading, track, and chorus. Her teacher describes her as bright, a hard worker, cheerful, and sociable.

3. **Reasons for assessment**

   A. List behavioral, emotional, social, academic concerns here and, when appropriate, identify the source(s) of information (e.g., "Ms. Miller, the librarian, reported that Jane seems to be isolating herself from her classmates during library group time"):

      1. Elisa expresses greater difficulty with memory and concentration, which have been confirmed via cognitive assessments with the Area Education Agency.
      2. She reports feeling fatigued throughout the day, despite getting enough rest.
      3. She frequently (> 3x week) complains of stomachaches that go away after a short period of resting.
      4. Over the past month Elisa's teachers have reported concerns that she is more withdrawn, tearful, and irritable during the school day. She tends to isolate herself from her friends in the lunchroom. Although she is eager to learn, Elisa is also "hard on herself" when it takes her more time or effort to complete a task or assignment than her peers.

   B. List specific problems in any of the following areas.

      Eating <u>No significant concerns</u>

      Medication or treatment <u>No significant concerns</u>

      Health concerns <u>Elisa often complains of stomachaches and fatigue</u>

      Peers <u>Elisa has become increasingly withdrawn</u>

      Physical activities <u>No significant concerns</u>

      Relationships <u>Noted above in regard to peers</u>

      School <u>Elisa is having difficulties with memory and concentration</u>

   C. Describe the details and context within which the identified problem(s) is occurring:

      Elisa is experiencing these difficulties throughout the school day, but they seem to get worse during the last hour of her school day (approx. 11:00 to noon). Elisa typically waits for the office to page her when her mother arrives, despite knowing that she will be there promptly at noon.

4. **Coping analysis**

   A. Assessment of current coping
      Briefly summarize findings from assessments, observations, and information obtained from interviews or other sources.

      The Coping Assessment was completed by three of her teachers as an initial screening tool. They report signs of general emotional stress, cognitive difficulties, possible pain, and social/peer relationship concerns.

      Elisa completed the Coping Checklist and identified a limited number of strategies that she has used since her illness began.

   (continued)

FIGURE 7.6. Sample coping assessment worksheet for Elisa.

FIGURE 7.6. (*continued*)

Elisa's teacher has noticed that in her creative writing assignments, she writes about her beliefs, feelings, and fears about her illness.

Her mother reported that Elisa is doing well at home. She is eager to catch up on schoolwork and does homework on her own. She has noticed fewer "social calls" between Elisa and her friends, but attributes this to Elisa's need to rest during what used to be her peak calling hours (6:00–8:00 pm). She also noticed that her "boyfriend" has not called in several weeks.

B. Initial hypothesis

Hypothesize about the possible reasons for the apparent obstacles to effective coping.

Elisa has experienced changes in her academic abilities and physical stamina. These have affected her school performance and physical performance (e.g., physical education and track). These were a primary part of her life as a preteen.

5. **Problem solution**

List potential interventions that appear to be appropriate for the identified problems.

- About my feelings
- My self-talk
- What can I do?
- Positive thinking
- Tease buster
- A lot on my plate
- Personal journal
- Masks

6. **Evaluation**

List tools or methods that might be useful for monitoring intervention progress and evaluating intervention outcome.

- Teacher will complete a summary of her weekly contact with Elisa's parents. With the help of the school liaison her parent's questions and concerns will be addressed and comments and suggestions will be incorporated to the extent possible.
- In collaboration with the school counselor, Elisa will establish goals for her weekly sessions. The counselor will complete a note on each session to further identify ares of need and monitor Elisa's progress.
- Selected coping assessments will be used to reassess changes in coping (e.g., teacher and parent observations, Elisa's self-reported coping).
- Her parents have scheduled a follow-up visit with the pediatric psychologist who worked with Elisa during her hospital stay. They have stated that they will provide any relevant information from this visit that will help us in further assisting Elisa. Also have the psychologist assess for Elisa's coping with pain and possible somatic complaints.
- A quarterly review and evaluation of the effectiveness of Elisa's Section 504 accommodation plan will be done.

Completed by: Miss Robinson/Mr. Blitz_____   Date: 1/15/03_____

Name: Elisa Smith   Date: 1/1/03

Date form completed: 1/1/03   Form completed by: Ms. Jones

Which of the following accommodations/modifications does the student need to be successful in the classroom?

PHYSICAL ARRANGEMENT OF ROOM/ENVIRONMENT

_____ Seating student near teacher

_____ Seating student near a positive role model

_____ Standing near the student when giving directions or presenting lessons

__X__ Avoiding distracting stimuli (e.g., sounds of air conditioner, high traffic area, etc.)

_____ Increasing distance between desks

_____ Providing preferential seating

_____ Providing opportunity for movement

_____ Allowing use of headphones to block out distractions

_____ Altering physical arrangement of room

_____ Reducing/minimizing distractions (e.g., visual, auditory, spatial)

_____ Seating student near positive role model

_____ Offering cooling-off period/place

_____ Allowing alternate setting/mode for speeches/presentations

_____ _Additional accommodations:_ _____

LESSON PRESENTATION

_____ Pairing students to check work

_____ Writing key points on the board

__X__ Providing peer tutoring

_____ Providing visual aids, large print, films, organizational outlines

_____ Providing peer note taker

__X__ Making sure directions are understood

_____ Including a variety of activities during each lesson

__X__ Repeating directions to the student after they have been given to the class; then have him or her repeat and explain directions to teacher

__X__ Providing written outline, listing key points and concepts

_____ Providing study guides

_____ Allowing for frequent conferences with instructor to check for understanding

__X__ Allowing student to tape record lessons

_____ Having child review key points orally

_____ Teaching through multisensory modes (i.e., visual, auditory, kinestetics, olfactory)

_____ Using computer-assisted instruction

_____ Providing a model or demonstration to help students; posting the model and referring to it often

_____ Accompanying oral directions with written directions for student reference

_____ Providing cross-age peer tutoring to assist the student in finding the main idea

_____ Underlining, highlighting, using cue cards, etc.

__X__ Breaking longer presentations into shorter segments

_____ _Additional accommodations:_ _____

ASSIGNMENTS/WORKSHEETS

_____ Allowing extra time to complete tasks

__X__ Simplifying complex directions

_____ Handing worksheets out one at a time

_____ Highlighting key concepts on handouts

__X__ Reducing the reading level of the assignments

(continued)

FIGURE 7.7. Sample accommodations checklist for Elisa.

FIGURE 7.7. (*continued*)

_____ Requiring fewer correct responses to achieve grade (i.e., quality vs. quantity)

_X_ Allowing student to tape record assignments/homework

_____ Providing a structured routine in written form

_____ Providing study skills training/learning strategies

_____ Giving frequent short quizzes and avoiding long tests

_____ Shortening assignments; breaking work into smaller segments

_____ Allowing typewritten or computer-printed assignments prepared by the student or dictated by the student and recorded by someone else, if needed

_____ Using self-monitoring devices

_X_ Reducing homework assignments

_____ Not grading handwriting

_____ Not requiring cursive or manuscript writing

_____ Reversals or transpositions of letters and numbers should not be marked wrong, but pointed out for correction

_____ Not requiring lengthy outside reading assignments

_____ Monitoring by teacher of student's self-paced assignments (e.g., daily, weekly, biweekly)

_X_ Arranging for homework assignments to reach home with clear, concise directions

_____ Recognizing and giving credit for student's oral participation in class

_____ Modifying expectations for assignments requiring speed and accuracy

_____ Providing alternative options for assignments

_____ Providing extra options for assignments

_____ *Additional accommodations:* _____

TEXTBOOKS/MATERIALS

_____ Providing tape-recorded books and/or modified textbooks (e.g., lower reading levels with the same information, when possible)

_____ Attending to arrangement of material on page

_____ Providing highlighted texts/study guides

_____ Using supplementary materials

_____ Providing large-print materials

_____ Providing special equipment/assistive technology

_____ Highlighting important vocabulary, specific concepts, names, and dates prior to assigned reading

TEST TAKING

_____ Allowing open-book exams

_____ Giving exam orally

_____ Giving take-home tests

_____ Using more objective items (i.e., fewer essay responses)

_____ Allowing student to tape record test answers

_____ Giving frequent short quizzes, not long exams

_____ Allowing extra time for exams

_____ Reading test items to student

_____ Avoiding conditions of time or competition pressure

_____ Substituting a project for a test to demonstrate knowledge learned

_____ Providing someone to record student's answers

_____ Highlighting key words or phrases

_____ Allowing clarification on test questions as long as explanation does not give away the answers

_____ Eliminating computer-scored answer sheets

_____ Reducing number of choices on multiple-choice test

_____ Allowing tests to be taken in a separate, distraction-free environment

(continued)

FIGURE 7.7. (*continued*)

_____ Grading essay tests on content only; not penalized for spelling, capitalization, punctuation, or grammatical errors

_____ Allowing dictation of short answers to essay questions

_____ Providing key words for fill-in-the-blank tests

_____ Providing large-print tests

_____ *Additional accommodations:* _____

ORGANIZATION

_____ Providing peer assistance with organizational skills

_X___ Assigning volunteer homework buddy

_____ Allowing student to have an extra set of books at home

_____ Sending daily or weekly progress reports home

_____ Developing a reward system for in-school work and homework completion

_____ Providing student with a homework assignment notebook

_____ Providing proof reader

_____ Gathering progress reports from regular education teachers

_____ Providing a visual daily schedule

_____ Using study sheets to organize materials

_____ Using notebook with dividers

_____ Posting homework assignment in the same place

_____ Providing procedure for finished work

_____ Providing sample of finished product

_____ *Additional accommodations:* _____

BEHAVIORS

_____ Using timers to facilitate task completion

_____ Structuring transitional and unstructured times/places (e.g., recess, hallways, lunchroom, locker room, library, assembly, field trips, etc.)

_____ Praising specific behaviors

_____ Teaching self-monitoring strategies

_____ Giving extra privileges and rewards for acceptable behavior

_____ Keeping classroom rules simple and clear

_____ Making "prudent use" of negative consequences

_X___ Allowing for short breaks between assignments

_X___ Cueing student to stay on task (e.g., using a nonverbal signal)

_____ Marking student's correct answers, not mistakes

_____ Implementing a classroom behavior management system

_____ Allowing student time out of seat to run errands, etc.

_____ Ignoring inappropriate behaviors not drastically outside classroom limits

_____ Allowing legitimate movement

_____ Contracting with the student regarding expectations and rewards

_____ Increasing the immediacy of rewards

_____ Implementing time-out procedures

_____ Using timers to facilitate task completion

_____ Offering choices for responding to classroom demands

_____ *Additional accommodations:* _____

School District: Landon School District

Address: 123 W. Education Ave.

Any City, IA 01234

Student: Elisa Smith **School:** Landon Middle School **Grade:** 7

Date of Implementation: 1/1/03 **Review:** Quarterly

Statement of Student's Disability as it Relates to this Plan: Elisa was diagnosed and underwent cancer treatment this year. Due to her extended school absence and intense medical treatment, she is behind academically and has learning difficulties.

Accommodation/strategy	Implementor(s)	Monitoring dates	Comments
Meet with school counselor weekly.	Counselor: Mrs. Jenks	Monthly	Meet as needed
Provide additional assistance with homework and past-due assignments, including (1) peer tutoring and (2) reduced assignments as necessary	Teacher: Ms. Robinson	This quarter	
Permission to take breaks during class or rest in the RN office when needed	Teacher: Ms. Robinson	Daily	No need to ask permission, just notify her teacher.
No rigorous physical activity (e.g., running)	Physical Education: Mr. Blitz Playground monitors	Daily	Elisa would like to moderate her own activity during recess based on how she is feeling.
Classroom accommodations to deal with memory and concentration difficulties	Teacher: Ms. Robinson	Daily	Repeat directions, give assignments both orally and in writing, break lessons into shorter segments.

cc. Parents/Guardians
Section 504 Coordinator
Educational Record
Principal
Teacher(s)

FIGURE 7.8. Sample Section 504 Accommodations Plan Form for Elisa.

Otherwise, confusion and rumors may circulate about Elisa's hair loss, weight loss, or school absence. Also, some information is needed to adequately care for Elisa in the school setting. It is very important for you, as educators, to allow Elisa and her family to decide when and how much to share about her illness. You can, however, explain which information is important for you to know so that you are sufficiently knowledgeable about Elisa's needs.

Elisa's peers will likely ask several questions about her, both while she is gone and once she returns. Table 5.4 in Chapter 5 (p. 66) provides a list of some typical questions children might ask about a peer who is ill. However, these questions will change depending on the age and gender of the peers and the type of health condition. In Elisa's case, it is likely that her peers will ask if her cancer is contagious and if Elisa is going to die. You will play an essential role in helping Elisa and her parents develop answers to these questions ahead of time. It is important that Elisa's parents have control over what you tell others about their daughter's disease. Figures 7.9 and 7.10 contain the consent form for disclosure of information and the parent's guide for how you should answer questions about Elisa's disease, respectively.

Your child has a medical condition that may affect him/her in school. Naturally, children may ask questions about your child's condition. You may wish to share this information with your child's peers and school personnel, or you may wish to keep this information private. There are advantages and disadvantages to each choice. Please indicate below whether you would like information disclosed about your child's condition. If you would like information to be disclosed, please describe your wishes below.

___X___ **Yes**, you have permission to discuss my child's condition with other school personnel and my child's peers.

_____ **Yes**, you have permission to discuss my child's condition with other school personnel but **not** my child's peers.

_____ **No**, we would like to keep my child's condition private. Please **do not** disclose information about my child's medical condition with anyone in the school.

If yes, please describe below what you would like disclosed.

Only give information to school personnel that is necessary for them to take care of Elisa. Tell Elisa's classmates that she has cancer, as we've discussed on the other sheet. Please do not discuss Elisa's prognosis with anyone or her physical limitations with her classmates.

Please describe below how you would like this information shared with others.

See sheet where we answered questions about her health.

Jill Smith	1/1/03	Mr. Blitz	1/1/03
Parent Signature	Date	School Official	Date

FIGURE 7.9. Sample Consent Form for Disclosure, signed by Elisa's mother.

Your child has a medical condition that may prompt the questions of other children. Below are a list of potential questions that children may ask. Please complete the form to indicate how you would like school personnel to answer the questions if they arise about your child.

1. What is wrong with Elisa_____? _She has cancer but it is in remission._____

2. Why is he/she sick? _Some cells in her body got sick._____

3. Can I catch the disease from Elisa_____? _No_____

4. Is Elisa_____ going to die? _The doctors are helping Elisa, and she's starting to feel better._

5. Can Elisa_____ still play with us? _Elisa can still do most of the things she used to do.__

6. Will Elisa_____ keep missing school? _She might miss a few days because she gets very tired from her medicine, but she won't miss as many now.__

7. Why does Elisa_____ look funny? _The medicine she took made her lose her hair, but it will grow back.__

8. Will Elisa_____ get better? In how long? _She's getting stronger every day._____

9. Why does he/she look so tired/sad? _Her medicine makes her tired._____

10. What can I do to help Elisa_____? _Just treat her like a friend, just like you used to.___

11. What should I do if other kids pick on him/her? _Stand up for her._____

12. Can I still be friends with Elisa_____? _Of course!_____

13. When is Elisa_____ coming back to school? _N/A_____

14. Should I talk about Elisa_____'s illness or not? _If Elisa wants to talk about it, but not too much.__

15. Why can't Elisa_____ play in gym class with us? _She has to let her body rest from being sick._

Other questions:
_Why doesn't Elisa talk to me as much as she used to? Because she is very tired from being sick.___

| Jack Smith | 1/1/03 | Mr. Blitz | 1/1/03 |
| Parent Signature | Date | School Official | Date |

FIGURE 7.10. Sample Answering Questions about Your Child worksheet for Elisa.

Assessment of Elisa's Coping

Elisa's coping strategies and their effectiveness could be assessed with various tools to be completed by Elisa and her teachers. Below are examples of tools that may be appropriate for Elisa, as well as what they might look like completed.

Coping Interventions with Elisa

Based on this assessment of Elisa's coping methods, it would be determined that she is engaging in counterproductive negative self-talk. She is also withdrawing from friends, to some extent. Additionally, it appears that Elisa is having difficulty expressing her emotions and finding ways to manage the stress related to her disease. From these findings, several interventions could be chosen that are likely to be beneficial in addressing Elisa's difficulties in coping. The school counselor could work with Elisa on these activities during weekly meetings. The counselor also could readminister particular interventions if it seems that Elisa could use a reminder or more practice in a specific area. Sample completed interventions and explanations are included below, as they might be used in the school setting.

I feel afraid when . . . *I have to go to the hospital.*
I feel disappointed when . . . *I do bad on a test, especially when I could do it better.*
I am really good at . . . *writing.*
I am ashamed of . . . *my hair (or no hair).*
I get excited when . . . *I can go out with my friends to the movies.*
I feel frustrated when . . . *I have to wear a mask all the time.*
Most of the time I feel . . . *bored.*
I am happy when . . . *I'm listening to music.*
I feel upset when . . . *I get in a fight with my parents.*
I am sad when . . . *I think about my friend who died in the hospital.*
I am calm when . . . *I am listening to music or writing.*
I was really mad when . . . *I found out I had cancer.*
I am thankful for . . . *my life.*
I am lonely when . . . *I am at school.*
I hope that . . . *my cancer never comes back.*

FIGURE 7.11. Elisa's About My Feelings completed worksheet. From Merrell (2001). Copyright 2001 by The Guilford Press. Adapted by permission.

About My Feelings (Figure 7.11). This worksheet was chosen to assess Elisa's cognitive appraisal and to help her articulate her feelings. Because Elisa is holding many of her feelings inside, this activity was used to help her identify her emotions and learn effective ways of expressing them.

My Self-Talk (Figure 7.12). There was some indication in the coping assessment that Elisa is saying negative things to herself when she is frustrated. This activity helped Elisa see how what she says to herself can affect whether she feels good or bad.

What Can I Do? (Figure 7.13). Elisa appeared to be having difficulty finding activities that could help her relax or cope with her stress, perhaps because she is not able to run or engage in rigorous exercise—activities she found enjoyable prior to her illness. This worksheet helped Elisa identify new ways to relax and cope.

Positive Thinking (Figure 7.14). Similar to the "My Self Talk" worksheet, this activity helped Elisa learn more about how she thinks and how those thoughts affect her attitude. She also learned how to say more positive things to herself.

Tease Buster (Figure 7.15). This worksheet was used because Elisa's parents were concerned that other students might tease her, especially about her hair loss. However, Elisa did not report being upset by any teasing.

A Lot on My Plate (Figure 7.16). This activity allowed Elisa to recognize all of the different stressors in her life, not just those related to her cancer. She also began to learn how to manage one stressor at a time.

Masks (Figure 7.17). Elisa did not want to draw the faces in the masks because she lacked confidence in her artistic ability. She did, however, seem to benefit from discussing which feelings she tends to hide and how she hides them. Elisa really learned a lot about herself from this activity.

Personal Journal (Figure 7.18). Because Elisa was already using her creative writing journal as a coping tool, we decided to use this journal activity to address her thoughts, feelings, and activities more specifically. Elisa really enjoyed this activity, because she was able to organize her thoughts and worries without having to share them all.

Self-talk is what you say to yourself, and sometimes other people, about yourself. Self-talk affects how you feel. When you talk negatively to yourself, your feelings will probably be negative, too. For example, when you say, "I will never feel better," you may begin to feel sad or angry.

Directions: Below are some examples of self-talk statements that kids say to themselves. Fill in a *Smiley Face* next to the self-talk statements that are positive and a *Frowney Face* next to the negative statements.

"I will never feel better. My pain will never go away."

"I can help myself feel better by taking a couple of deep breaths when I feel tense."

"I always feel so tired. Will this feeling ever end?"

"When I start to feel bad, I can close my eyes and go to my favorite place in my mind. When I do this, I notice that I start to feel better and I have control over how I feel."

You have the power to change your negative self-talk statements to positive ones!

My Negative Statement   My Positive Statement

I'm stupid now.   I'm more challenged by my
                                                     schoolwork than I used to be.
My friends avoid me.   My friends don't know what to say.

FIGURE 7.12. Elisa's completed My Self-Talk worksheet. Adapted with permission of the author from Clay, Harper, Lehn, and Mordhorst (2000).

Everyone has good days and bad days. Sometimes the bad days seem like they last forever. Some kids have found that when they don't feel good or they are having a bad day, it helps to plan what they can do to help them through a hard time.

Directions: Below is a list of activities that other young people your age have used to help them. Circle at least *three ideas* that you will try the next time you are having a hard time. Then share this list with your parents or teacher so they have a better idea of how to best help you.

(Write about it for myself (keep a diary).)

Talk with someone about it.

(Pray about it.)

Try to fix the problem.

Talk to my friend.

Watch TV or a movie.

Take a walk or a bike ride.

Tell myself I can handle it.

Cry.

Do something I like (a hobby or activity).

Sing.

Play a sport with someone.

Read a book.

Focus on the best way to handle it.

Scribble or draw something.

Write to someone about it (a letter).

Create calming pictures in my mind to relax.

Say positive things to myself.

Talk to my pet.

Spend time with my best friend.

Run or exercise.

Practice the thing I've learned to do to help.

Act silly.

Don't give up.

Relax my body.

Ask a friend for help.

(Listen to music.)

Think of all the things I can do to help myself feel better.

Ask someone for advice.

Other things that I do: _____

I like to write stories. I wish I could run again. I wish I knew someone else with cancer that I could talk to.

_____

It may be helpful to share this list with your parents or teacher
so that they can give you the help you need.

FIGURE 7.13. Elisa's completed What Can I Do? worksheet.

Did you know that what you think affects how you feel? Worrying or thinking negatively can make the good things about yourself hard to find. What worrying, angry, or negative thoughts do you have?

Directions: In the jagged shape below, write a negative thought or worry. Below the shape, draw a picture of you. What do you look like on the outside when you are having this negative thought or worry on the inside? Then, in the cloud, find a way to CHANGE and rewrite the negative thought or worry into something more positive. Again draw a picture of you. What do you look like on the outside when you are having this positive thought on the inside?

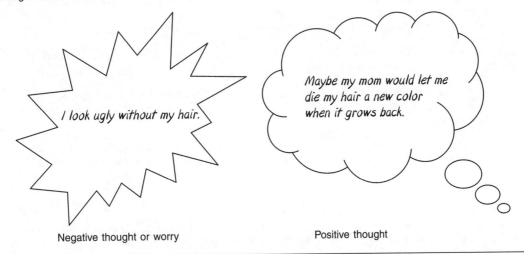

Negative thought or worry   Positive thought

FIGURE 7.14. Elisa's completed You Are What You Think worksheet.

Summary

This case example provides an outline of the resources and tools that may be necessary to help a chronically ill child negotiate the school reentry and coping process successfully. The individual needs of each child with a health condition will change, and it will be necessary for you to modify the tools to make them applicable to each child. For example, not all children need a reentry plan, because many are not absent from school for extended periods. Most of the information you will need to help individual children with health conditions have successful school experiences is provided in this book. However, we realize that you might need additional information to help these children, and thus the next section of this chapter examines additional resources.

Though everyone gets teased some of the time, and though teasing can be done in the spirit of friendship, it can also be just plain mean. When it's hurtful, here is what I think is going on:

People tease when they get a response . . . it makes them feel more powerful, and that's their reward. Teasing back doesn't do much good. In fact, it usually just brings you down to the same level as the teaser, and nothing positive gets accomplished. So, take away the reward by taking away the response that teasers learn to expect. Here's what I've found to be helpful:

- Try not to be drawn into the teasing.
- When it starts, make a joke of it or respond with a comment that you've practiced at home, or walk away while casually saying "Well, I'm out of here . . . better things to do to have fun" without appearing hurt. In other words, develop what's called "resilience."
- Think of yourself as a rubber ball instead of a glass that can be shattered easily.

Teasing also happens when people are uncomfortable or scared. If you're being teased because of a difference that others don't understand, how about helping them?

- Assume that they wouldn't tease if they knew more about the difference. You're the expert on it; you're the one who's learned how to live with it; so you're the one in the best position to teach them about it.
- Here's an example. Say your hair came out during treatment to get rid of cancer. That happens a lot to kids, and it's confusing and scary to children who don't understand, with your baseball cap on, walking into the cafeteria at school. Who should you meet but the biggest bully in school, who pushes your cap to the ground and says, "Ooh, baldy, what happened, cooties eat your hair?" You might say, "Nope, you got that one wrong! I'm taking some strong medicine that my hair just didn't like, so it took off for awhile. I wonder what color it'll be when it grows back . . . "

Directions: In the boxes below, write the things that kids say to you that are hurtful. Then write at least one idea on how you could respond to that statement the next time it happens.

The silly things people say	Tease busters (how I want to respond)
"Can I catch cancer from you?"	Say "No" (I do say that)
"Are you gonna die?"	"The doctors say I'm getting better" (I do say that)

Note from Elisa: *P.S. I don't feel hurt by things people say!!!*

FIGURE 7.15. Elisa's completed Tease Buster worksheet. Adapted with permission from Fleitas (2000).

Directions: Everyone (kids and adults!) experiences stress. This activity is designed to help you to remember this and to identify what brings you "stress."

Part I. List as many problems or worries as you can think of that other people you know experience. (Remember: *All* people experience stress or worry!)

money

getting sick

losing someone you love

grades

Part II. You will need an 8 × 10 piece of white paper, a few pieces of colored paper, tape, and markers or crayons to complete this activity. First, cut out, or ask an adult to cut out, 10 pieces of colored paper. Write a different problem or worry that you have on each. Next, draw a picture of yourself. Be sure to include *only* your head and shoulders on the page. Tape each "problem" or "worry" onto the self-portrait, stacking them on each shoulder. See how much you carry on your shoulders.

Part III. With an adult to help you, think about how you can solve each problem or cope with each worry on your picture. When you find a way to cope with a problem or worry, you can remove it from your picture, and if you want, crumple it up and throw it in the garbage.

Everyone feels worried or stressed at times, especially when we carry too much on our shoulders. When this happens, it is important to talk to someone else about our problems and try to find ways to cope with each problem or worry (one at a time!), so that we feel better.

Counselor Notes:

Elisa had five strips of paper on her plate, but stated that each was very "heavy." These included: her boyfriend not calling, losing her hair, worrying about cancer coming back, and arguing with her parents. She needed help determining ways to problem-solve. Even with help, Elisa did not find a solution to her problem with her boyfriend.

FIGURE 7.16. Elisa's completed Carrying a Lot on My Shoulders worksheet.

Directions: Sometimes people try to hide how they are feeling from other people. Using the circles below draw faces that show the feelings you sometimes hide from others.

Sad about my boyfriend

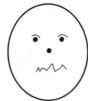

scared of cancer

mad at friends

Now draw faces that you use to hide the feelings you drew above.

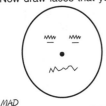

MAD

Nothing   Don't care about them

Counselor Notes: Elisa didn't want to draw faces today because she thinks she is a "horrible drawer." She did talk openly about hidden feelings, however, and I believe she learned a lot today. We used her thoughts about her artistic ability as an example of negative self-talk.

FIGURE 7.17. Masks worksheet for Elisa.

Name: *Elisa S.* _____   Today's date: *2/18/03* _____

Some of the **THOUGHTS** I had during the past week about myself, my family, school, or other things were . . .

I'm mad at my friends. _____

School is not as fun as it used to be. _____

Mr. Blitz is really nice. _____

_____

Some of the **FEELINGS** I felt during the past week were (circle the feelings) . . .

Happy	Sad	(Excited)	Lonely
Curious	Scared	Worried	Proud
(Mad)	(Tired)	(Bored)	Thankful

Write other feelings here: _____

Some of the **ACTIVITIES OR THINGS** I did this past week were . . .

Went to school _____

Did my homework _____

Watched Harry Potter _____

Babysat my little sister _____

Some of the **OTHER THINGS** that were important about this past week are . . .

Kyle still has not called!!! _____

_____

_____

_____

FIGURE 7.18. My Personal Journal for Elisa. Adapted with permission from Clay, Harper, Lehn, and Mordhorst (2000).

ADDITIONAL RESOURCES

In this section we summarize a school-based health and education program that was designed in New Hampshire as a model program for helping chronically ill students. We also outline two websites that we have found to be very helpful in providing information about children with health conditions. Finally, we provide a list of resources (books, websites, etc.) that you might use when seeking information about specific health conditions or about how to work best with the children and families who are struggling with them (see Handouts 7.1–7.3, pp. 169–171). We hope that these resources will be valuable as you continue to work toward helping chronically ill children succeed both in school and in life.

Health Education and Leadership Program

Project Director: Jeanne McAllister, RN, MS, MHA
Mailing address: Hood Center for Children and Families
1 Medical Center Drive
Lebanon, NH 03756
Phone: (603) 653-1419

The Health Education and Leadership Program (HELP) is a model multidisciplinary program designed in New Hampshire that attempts to "bridge the gap" between health and education for children with health conditions. Through the collaboration of schools, families, and local medical providers, this program helps to train school staff to respond to and help chronically ill children in a way that increases their chance of having a positive and successful educational experience. School principals function as leaders in training personnel and implementing changes that need to occur in each school. HELP is designed to assist school personnel in identifying and planning for children with health conditions through the development of 504 plans, IEPs, IHPs, and emergency medical plans. It is based on a family-centered approach and attempts to help schools adopt this approach as well.

HELP is divided up into modules of training and workshops, each addressing a separate piece of the health and education puzzle. The training begins with an explanation of why acquiring knowledge of students' health conditions is important—in the school setting, as well as describing the partnership between the different people involved in the community–school team. Several modules cover information about the needs of children with chronic health conditions and their families, as well as the developmental implications of those conditions. HELP training also covers what it means to be a "family-centered" program and how schools can incorporate this approach as well. Finally, information on school-related health laws and possible action plans for helping students with chronic health conditions is provided in detail. Tools and resources are available from the HELP program, and contact information for the program is available at the beginning of this chapter.

One of the greatest benefits of HELP is that it integrates the most important aspects of the lives of children with chronic health conditions: their health, their education, and their families. This program is an excellent model for how you, as educators, can be even more helpful to this group of children by working closely with the other important adults in their lives. We believe that you will find the HELP materials to be very useful. The available materials are relatively inexpensive and include a manual, multiple worksheets and forms, videotapes, and other useful tools.

STARBRIGHT Foundation

Web address: *www.starbright.org*
Mailing address: STARBRIGHT Foundation
1850 Sawtelle Boulevard
Suite 450
Los Angeles, CA 90025
Phone: (800) 315-2580

The STARBRIGHT Foundation is a nonprofit organization dedicated to helping chronically ill children and teens thrive as they continuously cope with the physical, psychological, and social challenges they face. STARBRIGHT projects educate, entertain, support, and empower children living with chronic and life-threatening illness to take back their childhoods. A number of resources is available for children, including:

- STARBRIGHT World, a private online community connecting thousands of children and teens who are ill in North America. This online site offers access to chat rooms with other chronically ill children, e-mail, bulletin boards, games, and information about health care conditions.
- Videos designed for preteens and teens are available. STARBRIGHT videos are offered free of charge to families of children or adolescents living with a chronic or life-threatening illness. Videos include *How to Communicate with the Doctor and the Hospital Staff* and *Back to School: Teens Prepare for School Reentry*.
- Links to other informational sites that provide medical information and online brochures that can be downloaded or ordered by mail from the STARBRIGHT Foundation are also included. Although these sites may provide helpful information to teens, parents, and educators, we cannot endorse the use of any specific website listed therein due to continual changes in the Web-based content of these sites.
- Educational computer programs are offered, including the *STARBRIGHT School Asthma Program* and *The X-men in Life Lessons*.

  1. The School Asthma Program makes available free copies of the *STARBRIGHT Asthma CD-ROM Game: Quest for the Code* and *Implementation Guide for School Use©* to school nurses across the country. *Quest for the Code* is an interactive asthma adventure game for children ages 7–15 that is designed for educational purposes. The *Implementation Guide for School Use* is a comprehensive guide that provides tips on ways in which school nurses can facilitate the integration of *Quest for the Code* into school curriculum for asthma management and how to use the game one-on-one with children who have asthma.
  2. The *X-men in Life Lessons* is a powerful educational comic book to help children (ages 9–17) who are survivors of burn injury and are coping with injury-related stressors. A Discussion Guide with tips and strategies for adults using the comic book with children is also available. The book is available in English and Spanish to burn centers, hospitals, foundations, support agencies, and camps for a nominal shipping and handling fee.

- Interactive STARBRIGHT Explorer Series® CD-ROMs are free of charge for children living with chronic illness, their families, and health care professionals. CD-ROMs are available for those with diabetes (ages 5–18), cystic fibrosis, sickle cell disease (ages 6–14), and kidney disease (ages 10–15).

Band-Aides and Blackboards

Site developer:	Joan Fleitas, EdD, RN
Web address:	*www.faculty.fairfield.edu/fleitas/contents.html*
Mailing address:	School of Nursing
	Fairfield University
	1073 North Benson Road
	Fairfield, CT 06824
Phone:	(203) 254-4150, ext. 2707

Band-Aides and Blackboards is a source of materials that may be helpful to children coping with health conditions. Its developer, Joan Fleitas, designed this site with children and teens in mind. Many of the resources available on Band-Aides and Blackboards are developed for kids by kids. The site offers:

- Information about chronic illness for children, teenagers, and adults on a range of topics
  - *Why kids get sick*
  - Questions and answers about illnesses
  - Helping kids who are being teased

- Information for parents and siblings
  - *Raising a child with a disability*
  - *How to talk to children about death*
  - *Through the eyes of a sibling*

- Coping tools
  - *Positive mental imagery*
  - *Humor*
  - *Personal stories from children and teens*
  - *Creative opportunities for children to submit personal writings*
  - *Poetry*

- Section just for educators
  - *Disease-related information (e.g., learn about sickle cell, HIV, JRA, cardiac conditions, epilepsy, blindness, cancer, cystic fibrosis, diabetes)*
  - *Classroom activities*

Figure 7.19 illustrates the site map for Band-Aides and Blackboards.

Summary

This section contains several resources that may be helpful in conjunction with this book. The HELP program is a guide to integrating a multidisciplinary approach to health issues for schoolchildren and their families. The STARBRIGHT Foundation and Band-Aides and Blackboards websites provide information for educators as well as parents and the children themselves. If you are providing these and the other resources (in the handouts of this chapter) to others, it will be important for you to become familiar with the tools yourself so that you can discuss and answer any questions that parents, children, or other educators may have. As educators, you play a vital role in providing information and support to all of those involved in the life of a child with a chronic health condition. We hope that the information and tools we have provided will help you feel secure, knowledgeable, and effective as you serve in that role.

Site Map

Band-Aides and Blackboards

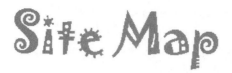

Child Content
What's it all about?

- Introduction
- If you have a medical problem
- Why kids get sick
- About special needs

Lots of Stories

- "Sally Goes to School"
- "The Nurse's Great Idea"
- "Kinka"
- Anthony: leukemia
- Jessica: neurofibromatosis
- Ashley: cerebral palsy
- Mysti: Pseudotumor ceribri
- Jess: lupus
- Trudy: Vater's syndrome

About operations

- Angela: cystic fibrosis
- Matt: spondo-epiphyseal-dysplasia
- Tyler: neuroblastoma
- Peggy: bipolar disorder
- Matthew: idiopathic juvenile osteoporosis
- Thomas: leukemia
- Trevor: Wilms' tumor
- Elizabeth: muscular dystrophy

What am I all about?

Teen Content
What's it all about?

- Introduction
- The good, the bad and the ugly
- Sharing secrets

Lots of stories

- Katie: Grave's disease
- Rebecca: scoliosis
- Alexis: CP, SCD, lupus...
- Adam: Crohn's disease
- Maddy: Ewing's sarcoma
- Dani: Rett syndrome
- Heather: rheumatoid arthritis
- Angela's essay
- Megan: arrhythmogenic right ventricular dysplasia
- Laura: aplastic anemia
- Georgianna: kidney stones
- Liz: arteriovenous malformation
- Emmah: bipolar disorder
- Natalie: Moebius syndrome
- Joe: adhd, asthma
- Stephanie: anklyosing spondylitis
- Lily: diabetes
- Kelly: fibromyalgia

Adult Content
What's it all about?

- Introduction
- About the title
- Clouds have silver linings
- Intro: "Sally Goes to School"

Especially for parents

- Parental permission
- The lowdown on teasing
- Raising a child with a disability
- Lynn's advice
- A lesson from Debbie
- A teacher's reminder
- A hospital orientation
- Tips for parents
- Communicating with schools
- A father copes
- Lessons in coping
- Parenting in the hospital
- The need to fly
- Guilt, the gift that keeps on giving
- Expert parents, robust resources
- Siblings in the storm of illness
- How to talk to children about death
- Chat with a pediatrician

FIGURE 7.19. Partial Band-Aides and Blackboards site map (www.faculty.fairfield.edu/fleitas/contents.htm). Reprinted with permission from Fleitas (2002).

HANDOUT 7.1. Reading List

- *Healing Images for Children: Teaching Relaxation and Guided Imagery to Children Facing Cancer and Other Serious Illnesses* by Nancy C. Klein and Matthew Holden
- *Guided Imagery for Healing Children and Teens: Wellness through Visualization* by Ellen Curran
- *Starbright—Meditations for Children* and *Moonbeam: A Book of Meditations for Children* by Maureen Garth
- Special Kids in Schools Series:
  - *Taking Diabetes to School*
  - *Taking Asthma to School*
  - *Taking Cancer to School*
- *A Tool Box for You: Activities for Helping Kids Cope with Serious Illness* by Deva Joy Gouss
- *Easy for You to Say: Q & A's for Teens Living with Chronic Illness or Disability* by Miriam Kaufman
- *Understanding the Child with a Chronic Illness in the Classroom* by Janet Fithian
- *Building the Healing Partnership: Parents, Professionals, and Children With Chronic Illnesses and Disabilities* by Patricia Taner Leff and Elaine H. Walizer
- *Meeting the Needs of Students with Special Physical and Health Care Needs* by Jennifer Leigh Hill and Ann Castel Davis
- *Chronic Kids, Constant Hope: Help and Encouragement for Parents of Children with Chronic Conditions* by Elizabeth Hoekstra and Mary Bradford
- *Coping with Your Child's Chronic Illness* by Alesia T. Barrett Singer
- *The Chronically Ill Child: A Guide for Parents and Professionals* by Audrey T. McCollum
- *Educating the Chronically Ill Child* by Susan B Kleinberg
- *Whole Parent Whole Child: A Parents' Guide to Raising a Child with a Chronic Illness* by Broatch Haig and Patricia M. Moynihan

HANDOUT 7.2. Web Resources

For School-Age Children

Kidshealth.org has kid-friendly information on all kinds of health and illness topics.

Band-Aides and Blackboards at *www.faculty.fairfield.edu/fleitas/contkids.html*

Bravekids.org provides resources designed to help children who are coping with chronic, life-threatening illnesses or disabilities. This site offers medical information on a wide range of illnesses as well as a directory of additional support resources. Information is available in Spanish.

For Teens

Encourage online.org is a place for teens living with chronic illness and their family and friends to talk, connect, and have fun with others who understand.

Teenshealth.org has information for teens on all kinds of health and illness topics.

Band-Aides and Blackboards for teens (www.faculty.fairfield.edu/fleitas/contkids.html) is a site that includes teenagers' own stories and poetry about their chronic conditions.

Chronic Illness Resources for Teens at *www.dartmouth.edu/dms/koop/resources/chronic_illness/ chronic.html* includes stories written by teens of their experiences with chronic illness.

HANDOUT 7.3. Resources on Self-Care

Websites

Following are websites where you can find additional information on self-care, relaxation, and general mental health issues.
- *www.healthy.net*
- *www.mentalhealth.org*
- *www.stressless.com*
- *www.ncptsd.org*
- *www.youthmentalhealth.org*

Books

- *Self-Care Now!: 30 Ways to Overcome Obstacles That Prevent You from Taking Care of Yourself* by Paul Salvucci
- *The Healthy Mind/Healthy Body* by David Sobel and Robert Ornstein
- *The Resilient Practitioner: Burnout, Prevention and Self-Care Strategies for Counselors, Therapists, Teachers, and Health Professionals* by Thomas M. Skovholt
- *Creating Emotionally Safe Schools: A Guide for Educators and Parents* by Jane Bluestein
- *Motivating and Inspiring Teachers: The Educational Leader's Guide for Building Staff Morale* by Todd Whitaker, Beth Whitaker, and Dale Lumpa

References

American Academy of Pediatrics. (2001). Medical conditions affecting sports participation. *Pediatrics, 107,* 1205–1209.

Americans with Disabilities Act of 1990, Public Law No. 101-336, §1 *et seq.,* 104 Stat. 327 (1990).

Band, E. B., & Weisz, J. R. (1990). Developmental differences in primary and secondary control coping and adjustment to juvenile diabetes. *Journal of Clinical Child Psychology, 19,* 150–158.

Banks, R. (1998). *What should parents and teachers know about bullying?* [Online]. Available: *http://www.edrs.com/members/ericfac.cfm?an=ED424037*

Boekarts, M., & Roder, I. (1999). Stress, coping, and adjustment in children with a chronic disease: A review of the literature. *Disability and Rehabilitation, 21,* 311–337.

Bossert, E., Holaday, B., Harkins, A., & Turner-Henson, A. (1990). Strategies of normalization used by parents of chronically ill school age children. *Journal of Child and Adolescent Psychiatry and Mental Health Nursing, 3,* 57–61.

Cassidy, J., & Petty, R. (1995). *Textbook of pediatric rheumatology* (3rd ed.). Philadelphia: Saunders.

Challinor, J. (2001, March). *Returning to school with a chronic illness* [Online]. Available: *http://www.tipsonteens.org/tips/march01.html*

Changing Faces. (1999, January 14). *Supporting a child with a disfigurement: A teachers guide* [Online]. Available: *www.cfaces.demon.co.uk/g6.htm*

Clay, D. L., Harper, D. C., Lehn, L., & Mordhorst, M. J. (2000, August). *Efficacy of the biobehavioral treatment for pediatric pain.* Paper presented at the annual meeting of the American Psychological Association, Washington, DC.

Cohen, M. S. (1999). Families coping with childhood chronic illness: A research review. *Families, Systems, and Health, 17,* 149–164.

Daneman, D., & Frank, M. (1996). The student with diabetes mellitus. In R. H. A. Haslam & P. J. Valletutti (Eds.), *Medical problems in the classroom: The teacher's role in diagnosis and management* (pp. 97–114). Austin, TX: Pro-Ed.

Davis, M., Eshelman, E. R., & McKay, M. (1988). *The relaxation and stress reduction workbook* (3rd ed). Oakland, CA: New Harbinger.

Education for All Handicapped Children Act of 1975, Public Law No. 94-142, §1 *et seq.,* 89 Stat. 773 (1975).

Education of the Handicapped Act Amendments of 1986, Public Law No. 99-457, §1 *et seq.*, 100 Stat. 1145 (1986).

Eiser, C., & Town, C. (1987). Teachers' concerns about chronically ill children: Implications for paediatricians. *Developmental Medicine and Child Neurology, 29*, 56–63.

Ericson, N. (2001). *Addressing the problem of juvenile bullying.* In OJJDP fact sheet #27 [Online]. Available: *http://purl.access.gpo.gov/GPO/LPS13593*

Fleitas, J (2000, August 1). *Rubber balls bounce* [Online]. Available: *www.faculty.fairfield.edu/ fleitas/balls.html*

Fleitas, J. (2002, February 15). *Yarden and his imagination* [Online]. Available: *www.faculty. fairfield.edu/fleitas/yarden.html.*

Heegaard, M. (1991). *When mom and dad separate: Children can learn to cope with grief from divorce.* Minneapolis, MN: Woodland Press.

Hobday, A., & Ollier, K. (1999). *Creative therapy with children and adolescents: A British Psychology Society Book.* Atascadero, CA: Impact.

Individuals with Disabilities Education Act (IDEA). (1990). Public Law No. 101-476.

Individuals with Disabilities Education Act, Amendment Act of 1997.

Juvonen, J., & Graham, S. (Eds.). (2001). *Peer harassment in school: The plight of the vulnerable and victimized.* New York: Guilford Press.

Lau, R. R., Quadrel, M. L., & Hartman, K. A. (1990). Development of young adults' preventive health beliefs and behavior: Influence from parents and peers. *Journal of Health and Social Behavior, 31*, 240–259.

Laundy, J., & Boujaoude, L. (2003, June). *Your child: Development and behavior resources: A guide to information and support for parents* [Online]. Available: *www.med.umich.edu/1libr/ yourchild*

Lazarus, R. S., & Folkman, S. (1984). *Stress, appraisal and coping.* New York: Springer.

Lipton, D. G. (2003). *Individuals with Disabilities Education Act Amendments of 1997. and IDEA regulations of 1999* [Online]. Available: *www.redf.org/idea10.html*

Lowenstein, L. (1999). *Creative interventions for troubled children and youth.* Toronto, Canada: Champion Press.

Meijer, S. A., Sinnema, G., Bijstra, J. O., Mellenbergh, G. J., & Walters, W. H. G. (2002). Coping styles and locus of control as predictors for psychological adjustment of adolescents with a chronic illness. *Social Science and Medicine, 54*, 1453–1461.

Merrell, K. W. (2001). *Helping students overcome depression and anxiety: A practical guide.* New York: Guilford Press.

Moos, R. H. (2002). Life stressors, social resources, and coping skills in youth: Applications to adolescents with chronic disorders. *Journal of Adolescent Health, 30S*, 22–29.

Mukherjee, S., Lightfoot, J., & Sloper, P. (2000). The inclusion of pupils with a chronic health condition in mainstream school: What does it mean for teachers? *Educational Research, 42*, 59–72.

Olweus, D. (1999). *Bullying prevention program.* Boulder: Center for the Study and Prevention of Violence, Institute of Behavioral Science, University of Colorado.

Phelps, L. (1998). *Health-related disorders in children and adolescents: A guidebook for understanding and educating.* Washington, DC: American Psychological Association.

Rehabilitation Act of 1973, Public Law No. 93-112, §504, 87 Stat. 355 (1973).

Ryan-Wenger, N. A. (1996). Children, coping and the stress of illness: A synthesis of the research. *JSPN: Journal for Specialists in Pediatric Nursing, 1*, 126–138.

Sampson, R. (2002). *Bullying in schools.* In problem-oriented guides for police series, no. 12 [Online]. Available: *http://purl.access.gpo.gov/GPO/LPS19843*

Sexson, S. B., & Madan-Swain, A. (1993). School reentry for the child with chronic illness. *Journal of Learning Disabilities, 26*, 115–125, 137.

Spencer, C. H., Fife, R. Z., & Rabinovich, C. E. (1995). The school experience of children with arthritis: Coping in the 1990s and transition into adulthood. *Pediatric Clinics of North America, 42*, 1285–1298.

Spirito, A., Stark, L. J., Gil, K. M., & Tyc, V. L. (1995). Coping with everyday and disease-related stressors by chronically ill children and adolescents. *Journal of the American Academy of Child and Adolescent Psychiatry, 34*(3), 283–290.

Stern, M. (2002). *Child friendly therapy*. New York: Norton.

Sullivan, K. (2000). *The anti-bullying handbook*. New York: Oxford University Press.

Walker, D. K. (1984). Care of chronically ill children in schools. *Pediatric Clinics of North America, 31*, 221–233.

Wallander, J. L., & Varni, J. W. (1995). Appraisal, coping, and adjustment in adolescents with a physical disability. In J. L. Wallander & L. J. Siegel (Eds.), *Adolescent health problems: Behavioral perspectives* (pp. 209–231). New York: Guilford Press.

Wallander, J. L., & Varni, J. W. (1998). Effects of pediatric chronic physical disorders on child and family adjustment. *Journal of Child Psychology and Psychiatry and Allied Disciplines, 39*, 29–46.

Walsh, M., & Ryan-Wenger, N. M. (1992). Sources of stress in children with asthma. *Journal of School Health, 62*, 459–463.

Zolten, K., & Long, N. (1997). *Helping children handle teasing* [Online]. Available: *http://www.parenting-ed.org/handout3/Specific Concerns and Problems/teasing.htm*

Index